A life turned
UPSIDE DOWN

by Nikki Hastings

Little Knoll Press

Published by Little Knoll Press
Third print run – May 2015

ISBN No. 978-0-9927220-3-6
Copies of this book can be obtained
from UK bookshops
and online from www.LittleKnollBookshop.co.uk

Printed in Great Britain by Hobbs the Printers
Totton, Hampshire

This book is dedicated to Leah and Megan

Nikki's diary entry - Monday, January 1st 2007:

'Happy New Year

Well this time last year we weren't even expecting Megan and here we are now, a family of four. I feel so happy and content, I think 'complete' is the word I need - I have got everything I've ever wanted and it's great.'

CONTENTS

FOREWORD
by Debra Stephenson

I had the privilege of meeting Nikki in 2013 at a fundraising ladies' lunch in aid of Lewis-Manning Hospice. I say privilege because it is always a privilege to meet someone who is courageous, determined and inspirational, especially someone who has the ability to touch your life through meeting them for the first time. I sat next to Nikki at the table and she told me she had been a patient at the hospice. She seemed fine to me. More than fine – she was bubbly, enthusiastic, giggly even, and I felt we were instantly friends. This was a woman who was very positive about life and therefore was great fun to be with.

During the event Nikki gave a poignant yet uplifting speech about her experience of cancer, as a sufferer of the disease, and as a fighter of the disease. She made the whole room cry and she made the whole room laugh – and she made a whole room full of friends. I was in awe.

How does someone who knows, as Nikki did, that their illness is terminal, find the necessary amount of strength and courage to look cancer in the eye and accept that it's got the better of them? Surely Nikki was one of these rare individuals that possess the knack of being able to look on the bright side no matter what life throws at them. Most people would be in a mess emotionally – devastated, depressed, angry or at least despondent – especially as a mother of two children, with so much to lose. How do you find the strength to cope in those circumstances? Surely it would take someone special to find the strength that Nikki displayed that day.

Nikki was certainly special, but in her speech she revealed that she had not always been so positive. She had been through shock, devastation and despair, and somehow found her way along a path to becoming the strong and courageous, positive lady who was standing before us.

Nikki elaborates on this theme in this book. The words 'searingly honest', sometimes overused in describing autobiographies, are nonetheless fitting for Nikki's account of her cancer ordeal. For the sake of others in need of catharsis, if not guidance on living through terminal cancer, Nikki has done a brave and courageous thing by sharing her own very personal experience. I am glad that readers will have the opportunity to get to know her through her boldly written and honest documentation of her difficult journey, so that they may be encouraged to move forward in life positively, despite cancer. Moreover, to see that it's even possible to have fun on the way, incredible as that may sound. Nikki's book is evidence that there is life after the diagnosis of terminal cancer and however much or little there is left, it's possible to live that life to the full.

If anyone was ever in any doubt as to why cancer sufferers need so much support outside of their treatment, this book provides necessary enlightenment. Nikki credits the people in her life that helped her – her family and friends – but her book also highlights just how essential the work is of organisations such as Lewis-Manning Hospice, Macmillan and Breast Cancer Care.

In *A life turned Upside Down* Nikki shares how she navigated her way through cancer from a state of shock, depression, torment and struggle, to acceptance and becoming the happy, strong, brave and positive lady whom it was my privilege to meet.

Debra Stephenson
Patron of Lewis-Manning Hospice

What can I say - one cannot read this book and not be moved - A very brave LADY.

ACKNOWLEDGEMENTS

Nikki's story starts with her terminal diagnosis and continues through the years that she thought she would never have. The subject is a difficult one, but Nikki wrote as if she was speaking to a friend, not asking the reader to be sad, or to be impressed, just to understand. She wrote the book that she was looking for when first diagnosed, one by an ordinary person telling another about her experience of living with cancer.

Nikki wanted to acknowledge in this book the people who gave her the chance to live a full life and to write. They are many, and if I have not mentioned some of you here, you will know who you are. Known to me are: her husband, Kev, her mum, Ann, her daughters, Leah and Megan, to whom she has dedicated the book, close relatives and friends who were always there for her, the staff at the Bournemouth Echo, who published her blog and sowed the seed for the book, the 'Once Upon a Time' writers' group, who gave her friendship and help with writing craft, the staff and fellow patients at Lewis-Manning Hospice and staff of the Christchurch Macmillan Unit and Day Centre, who provided wonderful care and solace during her illness and at the end of her life.

It is also clear that Nikki felt huge gratitude to the doctors, nurses and medical staff who treated her with kindness and the best medical care available at the time. She was in no doubt that this extended her life. In her book she describes her body's response to the different drug regimes. Whilst accepting that each person's response to treatment is unique, it is due to the sharing of information that treatments advance, meaning that the particular drug regimes that she describes should not be taken as a guide to practise in the future.

Since Nikki's manuscript left her hands, other people have helped to bring her book to completion; Kev and Ann by adding their words and the photographs, Nikki's Uncle Steve with his poem, Debra Stephenson in writing the foreword and Heather Freeman in writing the postscript.

This book brought together a lot of people in the making and it will continue to do so, adding to our understanding of terminal illness.

Jenny Knowles, Editor & publisher

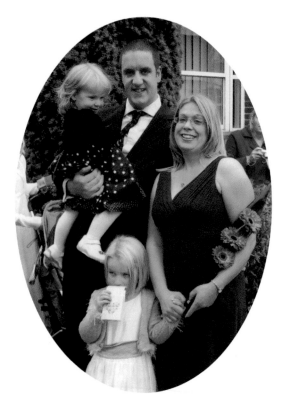

Nikki and family at Mel's wedding
October 2008

1

How it happened

The diagnosis of terminal cancer is the beginning of a journey – whether it's a journey to death or a journey to a new life, is up to the patient.

For two days after my sister Mel's wedding I felt as if I had a hangover. I knew I couldn't, because I'd only had four glasses of wine over the whole day, but a hangover was certainly what it felt like. When I awoke on the third morning with a strange feeling under my rib cage, I really started to worry. I wasn't in pain, but it was very uncomfortable, particularly when I breathed in.

As soon as my GP surgery opened at 8am, I was on the phone and managed to get an appointment for 9.20am. The children, Leah (four years old) and Megan (two years old), were due in nursery, so I didn't need to worry about childcare.

The doctor asked me what the problem was, so I explained the discomfort under my rib cage and the hung-over feeling of the past couple of days. He examined me and told me he could feel something in the area of my gall bladder. "You need to get yourself to the hospital," he said, "… and take an overnight bag – just in case."

On the way to the hospital I made a few phone calls. My mother-in-law expressed deep sympathy for the pain I must be in – she had experienced gall stones and knew what agony they were. At that moment it did cross my mind that maybe we were dealing with something else.

As soon as the doctor at the hospital examined me, he told me it was my liver causing the discomfort, and he asked me to tell him what I'd been doing over the past few days. So I told him about the wedding and the hung-over feeling. He asked how much I'd had to drink, but when I told him, he kept asking if I was sure.

He then asked about painkillers. I mentioned my hip, which had been hurting for the past month – I thought I'd pulled or twisted something when we had been to Legoland. I told him I'd been taking paracetamol for the pain. That was when he put the pressure on: "Are you sure you took the correct dosage? Are you sure that's all you had to drink? Are you sure? Are you sure?" I started to feel very confused and overwhelmed.

They decided to keep me in hospital overnight and do a scan in the morning. My husband, Kev, arranged for his sister Leanne to pick the girls up from nursery, so that he could stay with me through visiting hours.

The doctor told me he wasn't overly concerned, because I didn't seem to be particularly ill. I felt as if I was being a nuisance and a hypochondriac, and that feeling intensified when in the middle of the night I was woken up to be told they needed my bed, and so moved to another ward.

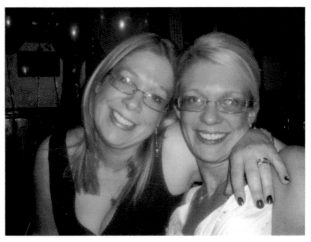

Nikki and Mel on Mel's wedding day, 25th October 2008

The next morning Kev took the girls to Mum's (where they would normally have been on a Wednesday, because I would usually be at work) and he went to work. He told me to ring him as soon as I had any news.

At about 10am I was taken to have an ultrasound scan. It

was just like when I was pregnant, except there was no baby to see. Not long after I had arrived back on the ward, three doctors approached me. One sat on the edge of my bed and took my hand in hers, one looked like Alan Carr (he did the talking) and another, Dr Tom, stood there looking rather awkward, but embarrassingly gorgeous (in a phwoar sort of way). The Alan Carr look-alike explained that they could see something on my liver and they needed to rule out cancer cells. I calmly explained to them that they must be mistaken, my thoughts being that my uncle had died of lung cancer only six weeks ago and it couldn't possibly be happening to my family again so soon. The doctor, who was holding my hand, squeezed it and told me to call someone to be with me, adding that I didn't need to worry about visiting times any more. They then said that they would arrange a CT scan for me, but it probably wouldn't be until tomorrow.

By the time Kev and Mum arrived, I had been moved to a private room and been offered a 'nice cup of tea'. I was very scared.

About an hour later, a porter arrived to take me down for a CT scan (the one they didn't think they'd be able to fit in until tomorrow). A CT scan involves having to drink two pints of water and then being injected with a contrast dye. I could feel the dye warmly travelling around my body, and when it came to my groin I felt as if I'd wet myself, which considering the amount of water I'd had to drink, I couldn't be sure I hadn't.

Shortly after the scan, the Alan Carr look-alike came to see me again. He said he wasn't a trained radiologist, but from what he could see of the scan, it certainly looked like cancer cells on my liver. He went on to explain that it was very uncommon for liver cancer to develop in a person of my age; it usually comes from somewhere else. He said that the CT scan had shown a small lump in my right breast, which could be the primary source, and also some areas in my bones. I told him about the pain in my hip, and he nodded.

A breast specialist was duly called to examine my breast. He couldn't feel anything, but agreed that what they could see on the scan needed to be further investigated. I was booked in for a mammogram and biopsy on the next day.

Dad came in on his way home from work to pick Mum up from the hospital. He arrived whilst the doctor was still with us, and he asked for things to be explained again so he could hear what had been said. It was helpful to hear the doctor go through things once again, and I think it helped it to sink in a little bit.

Mum and Dad then went home, and Kev went to see the girls and afterwards to go and play poker. Some people have commented that I was mad to let him go, but I think we both just wanted a bit of normality – I wanted a bit of space and he wanted to switch off for a while.

When they had all gone, I made some phone calls. I phoned my friends, and each time I told them what was happening, it felt a little bit more real. At that point I had absolutely no idea what was really going on.

Kev came back to spend the night in the armchair next to my bed. We talked about surgery and other imagined options. We had a lot of hope that this wasn't too big a deal.

The next morning I had my mammogram and biopsy. The doctor carrying out the procedure was lovely; she comforted me when I burst into tears, and told me that although it couldn't be confirmed until the results came back in a few days, she was sure the breast lump was the primary source of the cancer.

Back in my room, 'Alan Carr' discharged me home. He gave me a prescription for painkillers and an appointment to come to Outpatients on Tuesday to see a breast cancer consultant. I would get the results of the biopsy then and find out what course of treatment would be best for me.

Still clinging on to a little bit of hope, I asked what I should tell people. "Do I have cancer?" I asked.

He sounded sad as he said, "We're not considering anything else at this stage."

I was so pleased to be going home; I was desperate to see the girls, but also very scared. I didn't want to upset them, and I knew I would cry when I saw them. They didn't mind my tears; they were pleased to have Mummy home and gave me lots of cuddles. Leah tells me that she remembers Auntie Leanne picking her up from nursery and telling her that there was a surprise at home for her. The surprise turned out to be me, sitting in my usual seat at the end of the sofa. That seat now has to be my seat, I'm not allowed to sit anywhere else and if someone sits in my seat there was a time when Leah would have told them off.

It is nice that Leah has such a vivid picture of what was a happy moment for her. I hope it is a memory she can keep hold of. I have few memories from when I was that age; my most significant early memory was the day my brother was born. I remember waking up in my parents' bed, but instead of them being there, it was Granny. Dad arrived shortly after to pick up some clothes for Mum, to take to the hospital. I clearly recall him saying, "You have a baby brother." I was nearly five years old. Apparently, it was me who chose his name, Matthew – but I don't remember that.

That night Mum, Dad and Matt (my brother) joined Kev and me for a Chinese takeaway. I have no idea what I ate. It felt surreal, all trying to behave normally, but knowing that for us normal had just completely changed.

Over the next few days I phoned everyone I knew. I wanted to talk about what was happening and I wanted my friends to know. Maybe I was being selfish involving everyone at this stage, but it helped me to talk about it, and it also felt good having so many people rooting for me.

Those few days of waiting went by in a blur. Flowers and cards started arriving from my friends and family. Mel came home from her honeymoon and we hugged and cried together. Before I knew it, my appointment day had arrived.

No nonsense

The appointment was for late in the day, meaning I had to endure many more hours of waiting – waiting to hear my fate.

It had been decided that Mel would accompany Kev and me to the hospital. She worked as a palliative care assistant (end of life care) and so we felt she was qualified and would help us ask the 'right' questions. All the pamphlets I'd been given expressed the importance of knowledge, telling you to write your questions down or even take a voice recorder with you, so that you can go over what was said afterwards.

We sat in the outpatients' waiting room … the doctor was running late. Kev bought a coffee and paced the room, drinking but not tasting it. Mel and I flicked through the out of date magazines, not seeing the words, but needing something to do with our hands. After twenty minutes had passed since our appointment time, I decided to go to the toilet, thinking it would be sod's law if they called me in when I wasn't there. I was frustrated when my ploy to hurry things along didn't work. When we were finally called through, I was beyond nervous.

The doctor sat behind a desk, a student doctor sat behind us, and a health care assistant followed us into the room. It was a small room and crowded, causing an unfamiliar feeling of claustrophobia in me. The doctor didn't mess around. "Your results are back and I'm afraid, Mrs Hastings, I can confirm that you have secondary breast cancer. This means that the cancer has spread from your breast to your liver and bones."

He went on to explain that once cancer has spread from its primary source, it becomes incurable. He told me that there were treatments they could use to manage the cancer, but it would never go away. With that sentence I felt all my hope evaporate;

all my ideas of treatment and operations suddenly felt very naïve. He asked if I had any questions.

I felt a million thoughts going around my head, but all I could ask was, "How long have I got?"

The doctor replied with, "How long is a piece of string?" He explained that there are many factors and everyone responds differently to treatment, so he couldn't possibly comment.

The appointment was brief and I was told to come back on Friday to meet my consultant oncologist and discuss treatment options.

I felt let down. I thought I would be getting all the answers there and then. Instead I'd been told I had another three days to wait.

Kev drove Mel and me to Mum and Dad's house, where I fell into Mum's arms and sobbed and sobbed. "It's never going away; they can't get rid of it."

Dad and Matt were also there, waiting to hear the news. We all hugged and Kev and Matt went outside for a smoke. I hoped they would be a good support for each other, having been friends since before I knew Kev.

I knew other people were waiting for my news, but I couldn't bring myself to speak to anyone. I asked Mel to call my four closest friends, Cathy, Rhea, Keren and Chris, to fill them in on what had happened; everyone else could wait until tomorrow.

That night I wrote in my journal for the first time in about six months –

'I have cancer. I have breast cancer that has spread to my liver and bones. This means I'm going to die of cancer - they can't make me better. How the hell does this happen to a fit, healthy 34 year old? I've had no symptoms, I've been well in myself, a little tired perhaps, but you show me a mum of two under fives who isn't. Shit ... I'm bloody scared.'

In the days that followed the official diagnosis, I had time to reflect and take in what had happened. How does this happen to a seemingly healthy young woman? Did I really not know? Could I have picked up on the problem sooner? All of these questions filled my mind.

I thought back over the past year … it had been an incredibly difficult ten months. In January my Uncle Pete had been diagnosed with aggressive lung cancer. He responded well to treatment and appeared to be coping well with the disease, but when my parents were on holiday in New York, he took an unexpected turn for the worse. I spent time at the hospital, supporting my auntie and cousins in the absence of my parents. I will never forget seeing my dear uncle lying in bed connected to tubes, unconscious and unaware. Mel and I drove to Gatwick at 5am to collect our parents and tell them that they were too late to say goodbye – the hardest thing I have ever done.

Kev and I had also had our problems. His business as a bathroom fitter had begun to struggle. Cash flow became an issue and so we foolishly paid the mortgage and bought food with my credit card. Then when two customers didn't pay, one leaving us with a huge bill for materials, we were ruined. Not knowing what else to do, I phoned a debt management charity and was able to enter into a debt management plan.

The relief I had felt after that phone call was enormous, and when Kev told me he'd secured a full time management position with the company he worked for before he became self-employed, I thought our problems were over. I was absolutely emotionally drained, but convinced that things were going to get better. At the time I couldn't have known the underlying exhaustion that I continued to experience was anything more than a young mum struggling to come to terms with the events of the past few months.

As for other symptoms … I thought back to Rhea's hen night and subsequent wedding in the spring. I hadn't felt like drinking on either occasion … I'd had a couple of glasses of wine, but instead of feeling nicely inebriated I just felt tired. The same happened at Mel's hen night, four months later. However, I couldn't really have gone to my GP complaining of an inability to get drunk, could I?

The only other symptom I'd experienced was the pain in my hip. I first noticed it about a month before my diagnosis, after

8

Kev and I had taken the girls to Legoland for the day. Megan, at nearly two, was too small to go on many of the rides, so I had carried her on my right hip for most of the day. I assumed that I had pulled a muscle, or knocked something out of place, and ironically my chiropractor appointment was for the day after I'd been admitted to hospital.

I was able to reassure myself that I hadn't missed anything, that there was nothing I could have done to get an earlier diagnosis, so then, of course, I started to wonder if it had been my lifestyle in earlier years. I had been a good girl as a teenager and young adult. The church played an important part in my life and as a result I got married when I was 19 years old (good Christians don't have sex before marriage and we wanted to have sex!).

The marriage broke down when I was 23 years old, and I rebelled, I started drinking and smoking. I didn't smoke heavily, but I began binge drinking, working all week and then going out on Friday and/or Saturday night and getting drunk.

When I was 25 years old I went to university to study Social Science. A 'wise' tutor told me that most employers look for 2:1 degrees, because it shows the graduate was able to live a balanced life, whereas for most people to obtain a 1st involved so much studying that they found it impossible to socialise and relax. I took this as permission to party hard, as long as I handed my work in on time.

I managed it well; my flatmate and I went out clubbing two or three nights a week and sat at our kitchen table with a bottle (or two) of wine putting the world to rights on other nights. I suppose we probably had two alcohol-free nights a week, on average.

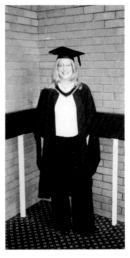

Nikki on graduation day, Brighton University, 2002

9

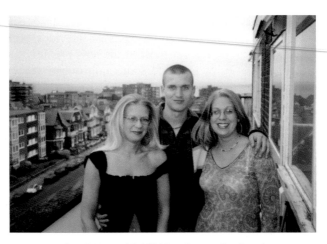

Mel and Matt with Nikki on her graduation day

Even when I finished at uni., graduating with my 2:1, I continued to enjoy going out and also drinking at home.

When I registered at a new doctors' surgery and told the nurse that I thought I drank about four bottles of wine a week, she was horrified. Her reaction prevented me telling her about the vodka and alcopops I also drank on nights out. At the time her response played on my mind, but I justified my drinking by telling myself that now I had finished uni. I drank a lot less than I had been doing over the past three years – 'baby steps'.

It was another year before I moved back to Bournemouth with my new fiancé, Kev. Saving for a wedding meant going out less, and once we were married we started trying for a family straight away, so my heavy living came to an end.

I will never know if those five years of drinking and smoking caused my cancer, but I had to tell myself that I couldn't dwell on it and I couldn't blame myself. For whatever reason, this had happened to me and I needed to deal with it … blaming myself wasn't going to help.

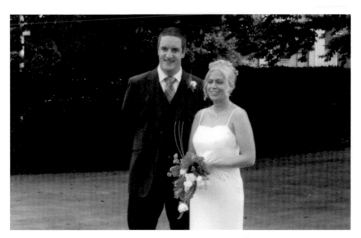

Nikki and Kev on their wedding day, 23rd August 2003

3

Chemotherapy

More waiting in Outpatients, Mel, Kev and I …

We were called through to meet Dr Hickish, a very quietly-spoken, gentle man. He expressed genuine sympathy for my situation and went on to explain the treatment regime he had planned for me.

I would have six sessions of chemotherapy, one session every three weeks. My chemo was to be made up of Taxotere, Carboplatin, Herceptin and Zoledronate.

Taxotere is a drug that works by preventing the cancer cells from dividing, therefore stopping the growth of the cancer. Steroids are prescribed alongside Taxotere to combat any allergic reaction.

Carboplatin is a drug which causes damage to the cancer cells.

Herceptin is a manufactured antibody, designed to seek out breast cancer cells and destroy them. Herceptin only works for people who are HER2 positive (between 15-25% of women diagnosed with breast cancer). This means that their breast cancer produces too much of the HER2 protein.

Finally, Zoledronate is a bone strengthening drug, also known as a Bisphosphonate. Bone cancer and chemotherapy can cause bone pain and weakness. Bisphosphonates can slow down or prevent bone damage. In some cases they can also help people with myeloma, secondary breast cancer and secondary prostate cancer, to live longer.

All four of the drugs would be administered by intravenous infusion over a period of six to eight hours, and the list of side effects was huge. I was to expect any or all of the following: my hair to fall out, nausea and sickness, fatigue, a higher risk of infection, bruising and bleeding, mouth ulcers, fluid retention, amenorrhoea (periods stopping), sore hands and feet, aching muscles, discoloured fingernails, high temperature, loss of fertility, loss of appetite, loss of taste or a metallic taste, itchy rash, hot flushes and heart problems.

I would need to have a CT scan and echocardiogram every twelve weeks to monitor the cancer and the condition of my heart, because Herceptin has been known to cause weakness to the heart muscles. Dr Hickish explained that the Herceptin and Zoledronate would continue for a year, because they were to help maintain the work that the chemo drugs had done. He emphasised that my hair would most certainly fall out, but the chance of sickness was low … and … if I refused the treatment I'd be dead within two months.

It was incredibly overwhelming; it was clear that these drugs were going to make me far more ill than I had been feeling up to this point, but to even consider refusing treatment was unthinkable.

I decided to ask the one question that was most important to me – "How long?"

Again I was told it was impossible to put a time scale on it, but if I responded well to the treatment, I would be well for 'some months'. Some months? What did that mean? However long 'some months' meant, it didn't sound very long at all.

For the rest of that day my mind was buzzing; every time I looked at the girls I cried, which of course upset them. I kept telling myself to pull myself together, but just couldn't seem to. I felt so angry, not so much in a 'why me?' way, but more about what I would be missing out on – mine and Kev's plans, the girls' teenage years, their weddings and their babies. Mum had been with me at both my daughters' births and I was being robbed of the opportunity to do the same for them. My whole future was being taken away from me.

I also felt angry about the effect my diagnosis was having on the rest of the family. Kev had withdrawn from family life. He had time off work, but didn't want to be around the house; he spent time fishing and playing computer games at his friend's house … he needed to switch off. He hated to see me crying and really didn't deal with it the way I needed him to, which then meant that he felt pushed away when I turned to cry with Mum.

Mum was running herself ragged; she was spending all day, every day, with me, looking after the girls, doing my housework, cooking for us, and then she was going home to run her house as well.

My Dad was a real worry. He couldn't seem to stop crying; he was never a very emotional man and I had never seen him cry before ever, yet now it all just flooded out. He saw a counsellor, but as he said to her, "What's the point of talking about it, you can't make her better and that's the only thing that will make me feel better."

Mel felt unable to do her job; dealing with patients dying of cancer was too much for her to bear, and she was signed off sick for several weeks, eventually returning to work in a different capacity, which caused tension among her colleagues.

My friends were amazingly supportive; I was overwhelmed by the cards and flowers that arrived daily, everyone saying they didn't know what to say, but that they were thinking of me.

Leah already spent two days a week in nursery, and Megan one day; the rest of the time Mel and my sisters-in-law, Leanne and Zoe (Matt's wife), helped out with the girls. I felt bad not wanting them around, but they exhausted me and I hated them seeing me upset. I decided that a small amount of quality time each day was better for them and for me, rather than me getting cross with them for being noisy, lively, normal little girls, or them watching me lying in bed or on the sofa, crying.

Eventually, Wednesday 12th November 2008 rolled around. On the day before, I attended Ward 10 for my pre-chemo appointment – an appointment where the nurse takes blood, temperature and blood pressure, and the registrar has a quick chat about your general health to ensure that you are 'well enough' for the chemo … how ironic!

Mum had volunteered to accompany me for my chemo session, and we arrived at 8am, armed with magazines and crossword puzzles. A nurse with a broad smile showed me to a chair and told me to relax. Not easy, as I was feeling absolutely terrified, the list of side effects was whirling around in my mind and, with my hand still sore from where they'd taken blood the day before, in a minute I would have to let someone insert a cannula (a needle) into my hand or arm.

I was told to warm my arm with a heat pad so that my veins would be easier to find. This seemed to work, as the needle slipped in nicely and my treatment was under way, slowly drip, drip, dripping into my arm.

I sat and watched as the ward filled up with other patients. There were six big chairs around the edge of the room, each with one or two smaller, plastic chairs for visitors. All the other people who were arriving for treatment must have been at least twenty years older than me; my eyes welled up as I suddenly felt very alone.

The day plodded slowly on. We were interrupted several times by various medical professionals; a Social Worker specialising in welfare benefits helped me to complete an application for Disability Living Allowance and told me about saving money with pre-paid prescription cards, as well as the Motability Car scheme and the Blue Badge parking scheme. I had no idea such things existed, let alone that I may be entitled to them. Then another Social Worker stopped by to introduce herself as the ward psychologist. She explained that she was there to talk issues through with any member of the family affected by a cancer diagnosis. She also gave me leaflets about other organisations, such as Macmillan, that offer all sorts of support. With so much more information to think about, my brain was fit to burst, but thankfully I had Mum there taking notes.

Finally, the fourth bag of medicine was put up seven hours after we'd gone through those doors and the end was in sight. A whole day had passed us by, I had been the first to arrive and was going to be the last to leave, the five other chairs in the room had seen several patients each that day, whereas mine had been occupied by me alone.

When we got home, Kev and the girls were waiting for us with dinner ready. I felt strangely alive and buzzing. I supposed that was maybe the appeal of recreational drugs?

Kev went to play poker that night. Of course I would have

rather he stayed at home with me, but I told myself it was important to keep things as 'normal' as possible. And because he went out, Mum stayed over, and she shared my bed with me, so Kev slept on the sofa when he got home. It felt special, being so close to Mum, and I know that although she frowned upon Kev for going out, she also valued that time. We lay in bed and I talked and talked and talked … everything that I'd been feeling came pouring out; my fear about leaving the girls, wanting to prepare things for them so that they wouldn't forget me, how I wanted to make happy memories and have special times with my loved ones. I'm sure it choked Mum to listen to me, but I was determined to get it all out and felt better for having done so.

4

Nic

Here the narrative is taken up by Nikki's mum, Ann Carter ...

I guess you could say I have had the 'perfect' life; married at eighteen years old to my childhood sweetheart, my soul mate, our only wish was to have a family and recreate the happy homes that we had both come from.

Tuesday, 30th April 1974, after an uneventful pregnancy and a relatively easy labour, our first little girl was born and we called her 'Nicola Jane'.

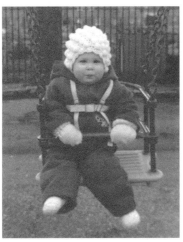

Nikki aged approximately 8 months

We went on to have another little girl (Melanie), and then a little boy (Matthew); our family was now complete.

Nic (as she was known to her family and closest friends) was the typical eldest female child; bossy, organizing, moody, feisty, stubborn, but along with these characteristics she was also kind, loving and very loyal. She was always in trouble at school for being a chatterbox, but she tried her best and worked hard, when she felt like it.

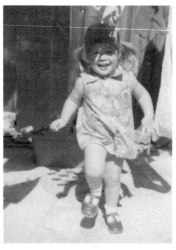

Nikki aged 2

We had lots of happy times with our young family, with Christmases, camping holidays, barbecues, and any excuse to get together with aunties, uncles and cousins (lots of them).

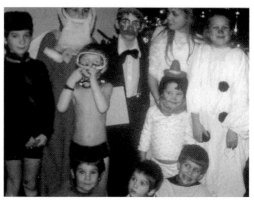

Nikki dressed up, with her cousins

We lived in a road with several other families, and weekends, evenings and school holidays were spent socializing and playing with all the other children.

Granny and Granddad (my parents), and Granddad Carter played a big part of weekend life, and Granny and Auntie Cilla helped out a lot when I worked part time.

When Granddad Carter's mental health began to deteriorate, the children were all aware of this, and their first brush with death was when he passed away due to Alzheimer's disease. Nic was fifteen years of age.

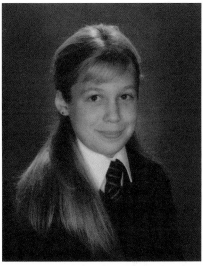

Nikki's school photo as a teenager

Throughout her childhood Nic had always been a 'joiner in', loving Brownies, Guides, and the local Chapel, which had a social group that she was a big part of. Photography was to become very important as a way of capturing special events and fun times for her. Her small group of friends remained constant from infant school, and they were still her close friends to the end.

Nic's ambition was to become a nanny. She attended

Poole College to achieve her BTEC in Nursery Nursing, and after qualifying, several interviews were lined up and she was offered a post, giving her the opportunity to travel with a family who lived in Chertsey. She was eighteen at the time and did not feel confident enough to leave home. I was very relieved.

She eventually obtained a job close to home, looking after a little boy, Joseph. I had back problems and was on sick leave from work, so Nic would often bring Joseph round to see me and we developed a close bond with him and his mum. When Joseph went to full time nursery, Nic went on to nanny for two or three more families, all of whom she stayed in contact with.

Romance was now in the air and she was married. Of course we thought she was too young (nineteen), but what could we say – we had married at eighteen. Sadly, the marriage failed, but that led to the next chapter in Nic's life, Uni.

Nic moved away to Brighton. She would come home occasionally and we would go and visit. She came to love Brighton as her second home, and this is where she made up for her 'lost' teenage years. She also made some more very good, lifelong, friends at uni.

Having achieved a 2:1 in Social Sciences, she started working with Adults with Learning Disabilities. She would become very frustrated with the 'care', which was all very well in theory, but did not work in practice and then the vulnerable clients were the ones that suffered. She did not hold back when fighting their corner.

Romance was in the air again and Kevin had moved to Brighton to be with her. However, he did not feel the same affection for the town and could not settle, and they moved back to Bournemouth. Nic began working for the Fostering Team with the local Council.

This was when she began to realize the importance of memories for children who had been removed from their roots. Moving to the Adoption Team gave her the opportunity to begin her 'Life Story' work, which became 'best practice' within the Authority. Research has shown that children who had access to their past, however harrowing, had a better chance of flourishing and not suffering from attachment or relationship issues in the future. Nic had always enjoyed craft and took easily to scrapbooking with the children's memories, and she was thrilled that this practice was to be rolled out nationally.

She became pregnant with her first child. When she went into labour, it became obvious that it was going to be a long hard struggle. She started off in Bournemouth Hospital and had to be 'blue lighted' to Poole, where her little girl was born 'flat', i.e. not breathing. Five attempts to resuscitate were made before her baby was breathing, and Nic did not see her for four hours.

Another little daughter was born two years later and her family was complete. Nic returned to work, and the girls went to nursery one day a week and I looked after them for one day a week – all pretty normal stuff.

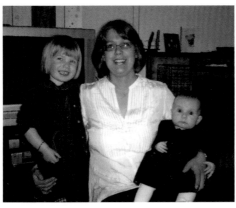

Leah, Nikki and Megan in 2007

Fast-forward to 2008; in January my youngest brother (Uncle Pete) was diagnosed with lung cancer, a massive blow to our whole family. He passed away in the September. Six weeks later, a few days after Mel's wedding, Nic was diagnosed with secondary breast cancer, no primary diagnosis, the cancer was in her bones, liver and lungs and she had no symptoms other than a painful hip.

5

Hell and back

'I had my first lot of chemo yesterday. It sounds so weird, talking about myself like that, it still hasn't sunk in.' – diary entry November 13th 2008

I woke up feeling sick and fluey. I had made an appointment at the hairdressers for the afternoon and, having made the decision to have my hair cut short, I wasn't keen to change my plans, so I ignored the advice of the District Nurse who had come to see how I was after my treatment. She said I should stay in and rest, but I didn't feel I needed to and I had to get my hair sorted out.

Having been assured by my consultant that hair loss was inevitable, I felt I had to take control of a situation that had so quickly spiralled out of my control. I had cancer, I couldn't control that, it had spread to an incurable stage, I had been unable to control that. I had to have horrible treatment that would make my hair fall out, and I couldn't control that either, but I could take control of the way I lost my hair. I could be passive and wait for it to fall out, bit by bit, clump by clump, spreading on my pillow each morning, clogging up my vacuum cleaner, or I could be brave and take charge of this terrifying situation.

I looked in the mirror at my gorgeous long blonde hair; I'd had many hairstyles over the years, long, short, blonde and coloured. Since having my daughters I hadn't had the time or money to worry too much about my hair, but leaving it alone had been the best thing for it and it had grown beautifully. Now I was going to lose it.

I decided I would go to the hairdressers and have a very short, cropped, pixie style (think Kylie post cancer) but when I sat in the chair and started to tell the hairdresser what I wanted, I suddenly changed my mind. I realised that this way I would be doubling the pain, cutting it now and then waiting for it to fall out in a few weeks. So I told the hairdresser to shave the lot off. He looked horrified, but seemed to know better than to argue with the crazy cancer girl.

I began to feel strangely liberated as my locks hit the floor, although it was a shock to see that the hair on the floor was in fact grey, not blonde. I had read about the way shock can cause such things and it gave me another reason to be sure that what I was doing was right – at least I wouldn't go grey. Somehow, I was able to look in the mirror at my face and not see my head. When it was over I looked at myself and saw my Dad looking back at me – I hadn't realised how similar we were before that moment.

I felt strong and proud of myself; I had done the right thing and, although I knew I looked shocking, I felt fantastic. I had taken charge and made a decision about what was going to happen to my hair ... this was a good thing, a very good thing.

I had decided that I was likely to feel uncomfortable wearing a wig, so I had sourced an impressive collection of hats, scarves and ski buffs to adorn my newly shorn head. I was taken aback by how cold I suddenly felt now my hair was no longer keeping my body heat in.

The feeling of euphoria didn't last long. When later that evening I was overcome with an intense feeling of nausea, I knew immediately that I had to call the Out of Hours Nurse for some stronger anti-sickness medication. I had to wait a couple of hours in extreme discomfort before a nurse arrived to administer the drugs. It was to be an injection into my buttock, and the pain was so excruciating as she hit the muscle that I wondered if it had really been necessary ... perhaps I should have coped? However, the nausea soon passed and I was able to have a good night's sleep.

On the next day I decided I would deal with any nausea with a strong mental attitude. There was no way I was going through the pain of another injection. That was until the vomiting actually started. I began vomiting on the Saturday lunchtime, and by mid-afternoon I gave in and agreed to a call to the out of hours team again. A different nurse came. She was abrupt and business-like, and I'm sure she thought I was a wimp for making such a fuss, but she did agree to give the injection in my arm. It still hurt, but was far more dignified than screaming in pain with my bum in the air. Trouble was it didn't work. I continued to vomit on an empty stomach for the rest of the afternoon and evening; I have honestly never felt so wretched.

Kev took the girls out for the day and then to stay at my Mum's overnight, as I didn't want them to see the state I was in. Mel sat with me, and when Kev returned they decided between them to call for help. A paramedic came and gave me a different injection; that was an experience I will never forget, lying face down on my bed with my trousers round my ankles and a not unattractive paramedic injecting and then massaging my rear end.

The injection eased the nausea and allowed me to rest. However, the drug-induced sleep gave me horrific hallucinogenic dreams. I awoke exhausted on the following morning, but managed to use the anti-sickness tablets that the paramedic had given me to put under my tongue to control the nausea.

Sunday was a slightly better day, until bedtime; that night I had chronic diarrhoea on the hour, every hour. When describing it on the telephone to Mel the next day, we came up with the expression 'anal retching' to describe how it felt to need to pass diarrhoea on a completely empty stomach.

By the Monday I was absolutely exhausted and very scared. Kev went to work, Mum came round to look after the girls, and I stayed in bed. One of my best friends, Cathy, came to visit and said that I looked 'in the nicest possible way' totally pathetic. That was how I felt, and obviously how I looked too.

The doctors at the hospital advised me to keep my fluids up and to try to change my way of thinking about sickness – with a tummy bug you would starve yourself for 24 hours and then gradually introduce foods again, but I had to continue to eat and drink as much as possible. Mel brought round some energy drinks which she had found in her office. I managed to force down half a vanilla flavoured drink at about 3pm, but at 7pm I knew I was going to vomit again. I leapt out of bed, collapsed in a heap on the floor because I was so weak, and threw up over my cream bedroom carpet.

This may be a cliché, but I felt like I'd hit rock bottom. I felt that I had lost all my dignity as my Dad (who had been sitting with me) ran from the room calling for Mum. Megan was already in bed, but Leah wanted to know what was going on. I was in a heap on the floor in a pool of vomit – I couldn't bear the thought that she had seen me like that.

Surely this wasn't worth it? For the first time since this all started I wondered if it would be better all round if I stopped treatment and let nature take its course. I didn't think I could cope with what the chemo had done to me … and the thought that this was just the first dose and I would have to go through this another five times, just didn't bear thinking about.

Thankfully, Tuesday marked a turning point. Still feeling horrendous, I phoned my GP. Miraculously, when I said who was calling, the receptionist put me straight through. I burst into tears as I told Dr Mitchell that something had gone wrong, I was feeling worse than I should be. He said he'd be right round and hung up. Ten minutes later he was on my doorstep.

I can't fault the treatment I have received from the NHS – especially my GP surgery. Dr Mitchell looked at me, listened to me and reassured me that everything was fine, and although it was awful, that was what chemo was like.

I felt better then, knowing that it was OK to feel as ghastly as I did, and felt that I would get through it, because others have and continue to do so.

I was prescribed some more of the steroid tablets that I had taken as a short course when the chemo was being administered. Dr Mitchell felt they could help with the sickness, could increase my appetite and lift my mood – all of which needed doing. I have no idea how long the sickness would have lasted if I'd just struggled through, but by the next day, the Wednesday lunchtime, I was feeling better, and that night I ate a chicken korma for my dinner.

So, a full week after my treatment, I felt better, had lost well over a stone in weight, been to hell and back, but had lived to tell the tale.

6

A New Year

'So, here's to 2009 – let's beat the odds and make it amazing.'
- Nikki's diary entry January 1st 2009.

Two weeks after my first dose of chemotherapy, my cousin got married. Claire is the daughter of Uncle Pete, so it was a very emotional day. He had been very involved in the wedding plans and we had all hoped that he would be there to walk his daughter down the aisle. After he died, Claire and her fiancé, Ashley, deliberated over the best thing to do. As everything was organised and they knew that Claire's dad wouldn't want them to change their plans, they decided to go ahead.

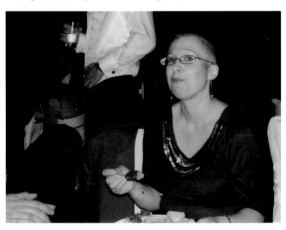

Nikki at Claire's wedding in November 2008

It was a beautiful ceremony, after which I went home for a sleep. The cousins, Mel, Matt and I, together with our spouses, Morgan, Zoe and Kev, were invited to the evening reception. By the time we arrived, the party was well under way, the bride was dancing in her trainers and the alcohol had clearly been flowing. I felt nervous entering the room. I was very aware of the way I looked, my trousers were falling down and, although I had bought a lovely scarf to hide my baldness, I suddenly felt that the scarf drew even more attention to me. I felt like a freak show, because of course everyone wanted to know how I was, how the chemo had been, to tell me not to give up, to ask how I was coping, how the girls were, etc. I know they all meant well and it was because they cared, but that night I just wanted to be normal again, to have the energy to join in with the dancing and the stomach for a few glasses of wine. The focus should have been on the bride and groom, and our host, my auntie.

Despite craving to feel 'normal' again, it soon became clear to me that I needed to accept a new 'normal'. Things were never going to be the same again. Following my diagnosis, Kev and I had sorted through our insurance policies, and when we discovered that the life insurance policy linked to the mortgage had a terminal illness clause, we tentatively put wheels in motion to make a claim. It took several weeks for a decision to be made, but a couple of days before Christmas we received the news that our mortgage was to be paid off. This meant that the doctor's report indicated a strong likelihood that I would be dead within twelve months. I felt shell-shocked; financially it was amazing, it meant we would be able to enjoy the time I did have left without money worries, but it really brought home the fact that I was dying. After struggling with financial problems for so long, we now had more than we knew what to do with, as well as clearing the mortgage there was also a couple of thousand left over.

It felt wrong that we were still in a lot of debt, but had this extra money. However, I didn't want to have to hand it over, I wanted to be able to enjoy it. I nervously telephoned the debt management company, who told me that as we weren't due a review yet, and considering our circumstances, she wouldn't record the call I had made. I felt very relieved and hugely grateful to that lady.

I did some last minute, extra shopping, and that Christmas

we celebrated in style. I was sure it was to be my last Christmas and so I wanted it to be one to remember. The children had a wonderful time … so many presents! I bought Leah a 'kiddy' camera in the hope that it would encourage a love of photography to equal mine. Megan wanted a camera too, but I think that was more about wanting the same as Leah, than a desire to develop her own photography skills. For the adults, the festive season was poignant – we wanted it to be special, but all knew that it would almost certainly be my last. I found myself welling up on several occasions, just watching the girls playing happily, and dwelling on what I would miss out on in future years. It was a truly heart-breaking time.

New Year brought similar emotions; we celebrated at Mum and Dad's. I had my third session of chemo during the day of New Year's Eve and so was lively and buzzing during the evening. We spent the time playing board games and drinking champagne. It was a bit of a house full, because as well as myself, Kev and the girls, Mel, Morgan and Dan, Matt, Zoe, and their boys Jay and Leo, as well as Morgan's brother, Corin, also joined us. At midnight we all raised our glasses to 'Beating the odds and making 2009 an amazing year'.

7

More changes

And so, into 2009 we went. We soon got used to the new routine created by my three weekly chemo cycle.

Week one would be a write off. I was very relieved that the steroids worked in keeping the sickness under control, and I didn't have to go through the experience of that first dose again. However, I did feel extreme fatigue – a tiredness that no amount of sleep would relieve. I spent most of week one in bed, either dozing or sleeping deeply.

Week two would be better; although I would need an afternoon nap of around two hours, I was able to see friends for coffee, maybe go for a short walk, etc.

By week three, I would feel a lot better and so would try to get out and about more. We planned special treats for week three for two reasons: to give me something to look forward to when it all felt too much, and to make happy memories for the girls and other loved ones. The problem with that was I would feel under tremendous pressure to make sure we all enjoyed ourselves. Kev and I had some really stinking rows on what were supposed to be 'special days', because we were tense and therefore snappy with each other.

I was very aware that people felt awkward around me and I worried about saying the wrong thing. I tried desperately not to make things difficult, but there were a couple of occasions when I did get upset. One friend exclaimed with excitement about how lucky we were to have had our mortgage paid off; I regretted my response of "Well, if you consider a terminal diagnosis to be lucky, then yes, I suppose we are." It wasn't fair of me and I knew she meant no harm, but I couldn't believe how insensitive her comment had been.

Another time, we were at my in-laws and I was complaining about some bad behaviour of the girls. Leanne told me to wait until they were teenagers, and raised her eyebrows to indicate that her older children were much harder work now that they were teenagers. My eyes welled up and I had to leave the room. I was desperate to know what my girls would be like as teenagers and I was going to miss it. I felt terrible for making Leanne feel bad. I realised then that I needed to toughen up if I wanted people to feel relaxed and able to be 'normal' around me.

I also realised early on that I needed to be more sensitive about other people's feelings. I took to making some inappropriate comments about my situation and it made people very uncomfortable. Mum, Mel and I treated ourselves to a theatre break in London. On the night we arrived, we were in our hotel room getting ready to go out and Mum asked if anyone had any hairspray. I quipped, "Hold on, let me get mine. Oh no, I have no hair." before laughing quite hysterically. Mum looked mortified and apologised profusely. I told her not to worry, that I had been joking, but I wished my way of trying to lighten the situation hadn't caused upset.

Another time, after picking Kev's wet towel up off the bedroom floor, again, I told him, "I'll be dead soon, then you can leave your towels where you like, but in the meantime please pick up after yourself." Kev walked away from me without saying anything, but not before I saw the tears in his eyes. Later, when we talked about it, I explained it was just my way of trying to make this awful situation bearable. I acknowledged though, that it had been insensitive of me and really not funny.

Trying to get used to my changing body image was a further challenge. Having lost so much weight during those first couple of chemo cycles, I'm ashamed to admit that my skeletal form thrilled me in a perverse way. I have never officially suffered an eating disorder, but there have been times in my life when my relationship with food has been far from healthy. When my first marriage broke up, I took comfort eating to a whole new level, eating tubs of ice cream and piling on the pounds. About a year later I suffered a serious bout of gastroenteritis, when I lost around a stone and my appetite diminished. Even when I was fully recovered, I didn't return to my previous eating habits. I started exercising and became obsessive. I lost three stone in three months, and for the next five years I ate very little and exercised a lot. I weighed myself two or three times a day and panicked if I put on weight.

When I was pregnant with Leah, I happily embraced the idea of 'eating for two' and after she'd been born, I accepted that my size 8 figure was probably a thing of the past. When Leah was a year old, I was pleased to be able to buy a flattering pair of size 12 trousers. Two months later I was pregnant again and the trousers went in the drawer to give me an aim when baby number two was older. I dug them out for my cousin's wedding and was outwardly horrified, but a little bit smug, that they now fell down.

In the January sales I spent my Christmas money on new clothes. Buying a new pair of size 8 jeans felt like the silver lining of my very black cloud. Thankfully, I didn't throw out my bigger clothes, because I hadn't taken into consideration the effect the steroids would have on my body. I turned into an eating machine and quickly replaced the weight that I had lost … and then some. By March I was a bloated size 16, bigger than I had been in many years. It was hard to deal with and one of the contributing factors to the depression that I soon developed.

Having finished the six doses of chemotherapy, I had a CT scan and Dr Hickish told me how pleased he was with the way the treatment had worked. The tumour in my breast had completely gone, as had the tumour in my lung. The cancer in my liver and bones remained stable. I felt overwhelmed and confused; I didn't know there had been a tumour in my lung, so that had come as a shock, and the irony that if the lump in my breast had been discovered before it had spread, I would now be clear of cancer wasn't lost on me. Dr Hickish explained that I would have another scan in three months' time, and in the meantime I was to go away and enjoy myself.

I really didn't know how to 'Go away and enjoy myself'. So much had happened in the last five months, and my life had changed beyond recognition. During my treatment we had got used to our new routine and now that was changing again. I had lost all my independence and felt very scared at the idea of trying to regain it. Everybody kept telling me what fantastic news it was that the chemo had done its job, but all I wanted to do was cry, and shout, "But I've still got bloody cancer, that's not changed."

I tried so hard to put on a brave face, because I was aware that when my spirits were high the people around me found things easier, but I couldn't control the crying. I wanted to be brave, but couldn't help but feel life would be so much easier for everyone if I stopped fighting and let nature take its course, and then everyone could move on and start their new lives without me. It scared me to realise that I was distancing myself from the girls, withdrawing emotionally. It was like I was trying not to care, because it hurt too much. It hurt too much to think of leaving them, so if I stopped caring it would hurt less. My emotions were all over the place and I was a mess.

I spoke to Dr Mitchell (my GP) and he prescribed anti-depressants. I was reluctant to take them, but acknowledged that I really had no choice. He also referred me to Nicky Ford, Macmillan's clinical psychologist, and just talking things through with her made a real difference. She helped me realise that my feelings were completely normal; talking and crying with her helped to get my thoughts in order and I didn't worry about upsetting her in the way I did about my Mum or Mel, because she didn't care about me in the way they did. So the next chapter in my journey involved regular counselling, lots of sleeping and trying to accept yet another normal.

8

A new arrival

Around the time my treatment ended, Mel announced her pregnancy. I was so excited and pleased that things seemed to be working out for her. She already had a thirteen year old daughter from a previous relationship and we were all happy that Mel and Morgan were to have a baby of their own, and that Dannielle was no longer to be an only child. It was such good news for my family, something positive for us to focus on, and for me it gave me another reason to keep fighting – to meet my new niece or nephew.

However, I still experienced sad feelings, I felt sad that I wouldn't be as big a part of this new baby's life as I have been in Dannielle's, and as Mel has been for Leah and Megan. The spiritual part of me also wondered if this baby was to be my replacement in the world. I remember as a child being told, and comforted by the idea, that old people have to die to make room for new babies. I was now twisting that idea and convincing myself that I would have to die for this baby to be born. I felt angry with myself for not being able to fully enjoy what I knew was a very special time. I talked it all through with Nicky Ford and she helped me put things into perspective; my feelings were perfectly natural and so I was to acknowledge how I felt and then move on. I don't know what will happen in the future, I don't know how long I will be here – just like everyone else, she helped me to embrace the present, that I'm here now, here to support Mel and to enjoy this special time.

When Thom Nicholas arrived it was a very emotional time for me. I was so touched that they had used my name for his middle name, and I will always appreciate the way Mel, Morgan and Dan shared Thom with me. I was allowed lots of special cuddles and they didn't once make me feel that I was being a nuisance when I felt I needed time with their baby. I can't explain that need: perhaps it was because Thom was so pure and innocent, there was no such thing as cancer in his world, perhaps it was because I'd thought I'd never meet him, so I wanted to soak him up as much as possible now that I had, perhaps it was because I wanted to do all my bonding now in case I didn't get the chance in the future … or maybe it was more simple than that, maybe I felt I could play 'the cancer card' and get away with demanding as many cuddles as I wanted.

Having completed my treatment and had a good scan I felt grateful that the chemo had been worthwhile. The fatigue continued for many months after the treatment ended, as did other side effects, such as nausea, metallic and dry mouth, blood/mucus clots in my nose, weak finger nails and leg ache. I also had to attend regular hospital appointments for the Herceptin and Zoledronate that I was still taking, and as a result I didn't feel able to return to work.

Thankfully, my employers, Bournemouth Borough Council, were very supportive and understanding. I received full pay for the first six months of illness and half pay for six months after that. I felt the time and the lack of money worries enabled me to enjoy my family and to prepare things for the time when I'm gone.

The first thing I needed to do was talk to my will advisor. Kev and I made wills when we bought the flat, a basic will that left all our estate to one another. Since my diagnosis though, I had been wondering what would happen to my share of the property if Kev were to remarry and have more children. Those children would be just as important to him as Leah and Megan, but they'd be nothing to me, why should they stand to inherit my half of this property? It turned out I was right and it was very simple to change my will, leaving my half of our joint estate to Leah and Megan, and naming Kev as a 'Living Tennant' so they couldn't turf him out when they turned eighteen. It was a difficult decision to make as I worried that Kev would think I didn't trust him to look after the girls' welfare. I know he would never intentionally do anything to jeopardise their interests, but if in the future he were to become mixed up in a messy divorce, it may be taken out of his control. This way I felt I was doing my bit to protect my babies. Thankfully, Kev could see my point of view and supported what I did.

I spent time going through old photographs and diaries. I have kept a diary on and off since I was ten years old. These books contain pages and pages of teenage angst, falling in love for the first time, and the second time, my first marriage and subsequent divorce ... and then the rebel years. Sitting reading those volumes made me cringe. I have never regretted anything I have done in my life, thinking that each experience has made me the person I am today – however my lifestyle at university was not a great example to my two impressionable young girls. The thought of Leah and Megan reading about those times without me there to explain it to them, worried me, and so one afternoon I burnt the diaries from 1997 to 2002. In hindsight I think I was a little ruthless and perhaps I should have produced edited versions before the big bonfire, but I did what I thought was right at the time, when I was expecting things to be over much sooner.

Having destroyed those old journals, I was now turning to my current journal more and more. I was producing pages and pages of my feelings, my fears for the future and the things I hoped to achieve before I died. I was aware I had changed the way I wrote, I was now writing with the expectation that my words would be read by my daughters and probably by Kev, Mum and Mel before them. I suppose when you write a diary you know there's a chance it will be read by someone in the future, but this felt more immediate and direct. I felt sad that my writing was being almost censored by my future audience and I was careful to write about each girl equally, with equal measures of positives and negatives. Instead of pouring out anger towards Kev when he had upset me, I tried to be understanding and forgiving, so that I didn't say anything that would hurt him once I was gone.

I wondered if accepting death was the same as giving up the hope to continue living. I had been told I had months to live. I needed to accept that, but could never give up the hope that I would have longer. In some ways I was blessed; we all know we're going to die; I just happened to know that for me it would be sooner rather than later. I felt lucky I had the opportunity to prepare and leave some sort of legacy.

I have always been a bit of a control freak and so it made sense for me to want to plan my funeral. I put a lot of thought into it and wanted to make the right decision about the girls. Between us, Mum (because Kev couldn't talk about it) and I came up with the plan that there would be a ceremony at the crematorium, strictly for adults only and then afterwards a child-friendly memorial service in a hall somewhere. I chose the readings and music I wanted, I spoke to Cathy and asked her how she would feel about reading the verse she had read at mine and Kev's wedding. I was touched that she agreed, but I made it clear that I wouldn't be offended if when the time came she felt she couldn't do it.

Having planned my funeral, I then sat down and wrote letters 'To be read on the event of my death'. I wrote to Mum, Dad, Mel, Matt, and to some of my closest friends. I didn't say anything they didn't already know, but I wanted them to have a written record of how much I loved them and how much they meant to me.

Doing these things felt very cathartic, I felt I was prepared, and so each time I had a scan that showed everything was stable, I felt confused, it didn't make sense to me. I had been told I had months, and yet three monthly periods would pass and I kept being told there was no change – how could that be? I had a scan every twelve weeks, and the week leading up to the scan I would develop aches and pains, which proved to be psychosomatic. On the other hand, occasionally the scans showed things I wasn't expecting. One afternoon Megan was sat on my lap playing, when she threw herself backwards. I grabbed her and a terrible shooting pain went through my shoulder; it brought tears to my eyes. I called Kev at work and told him he needed to come home and take me to hospital. Within about five minutes the pain had subsided, so I phoned Kev back to tell him not to worry and forgot all about it.

My next scan, about three weeks later showed I had fractured a bone in my shoulder. Dr Hickish explained that the pain had been masked by the painkillers I was already taking for the cancer pain. He told to me to make sure I had plenty of Oramorph (liquid morphine) at home, because I may experience occasional breakthrough pain. He explained that because I had bone metastases in my shoulder the fracture would never heal and would now always be a weakness. I felt quite freaked out by this; knowing how easily it had happened, I began to imagine all sorts of injuries and realised that there are more consequences of cancer than I had first appreciated. Having said that, I have only had one further injury since the shoulder, and that is a cracked rib. Again this showed up on a scan and I have no idea how it happened. These injuries mean I have no chance of ever being able to reduce the amount of pain relief I'm on.

9

Another holiday, Mummy?

And so, to get on with enjoying ourselves …

Because we had some money left from paying the mortgage, we booked a short break to Centre Parcs. We went with our friends, Rik & Gemma, and their son, Sam. It was a lovely holiday; I hired a mobility scooter to get around and experienced my first spa and massage. I had spoken to Dr Hickish about having massages, because I'd read that some aromatherapy oils and massage techniques can have a negative effect on cancer patients by interfering with treatment or by moving the cancer cells around the body. Dr Hickish felt that the benefits I'd receive from a relaxing massage would far outweigh any potential risk, and so began my happy relationship with complementary therapies. The holiday was fantastic – real quality, family time. I made sure we took lots of photos and that I wasn't always the one behind the camera.

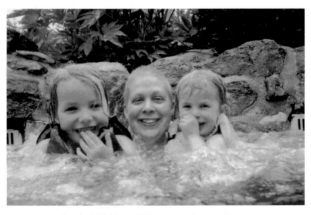

Leah, Nikki and Megan at Centre Parcs

When we came home, we raved about the trip so much that Mum and Dad encouraged us to take advantage of the discount offered if you book to go again within a few days of the end of your holiday. Due to my CT scans we lived our lives in three month chunks, not wanting to make plans beyond the next scan, in case it was bad news, so our next trip to Centre Parcs was booked for a month after our first.

Before we went back to Centre Parcs, I celebrated my 35th birthday and, because I was so sure it was going to be my last, I wanted to celebrate in style. I booked the hall where Kev and I had held our wedding reception and invited everyone I knew.

On May 1st 2009, one hundred and thirty of my closest family and friends (we have a big family) gathered to make my birthday the best ever. From somewhere I found enough energy to dance to all my favourite songs … I particularly remember standing with my arms round Ross' shoulders and us belting out Bon Jovi's 'Livin on a Prayer', waving our arms and trying to do a 'rocker' style dance. My nephew, Jay, and some of Kev's friends put on an impromptu 'Street Dance' performance, showing off their moves, and I posed for photos with everyone so that there were lasting memories of a very special, emotional night.

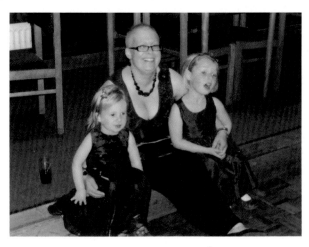

Megan, Nikki and Leah at Nikki's 35th birthday party

39

So, off to Centre Parcs again, and Mum and Dad came with us this time. I had been a bit concerned about Mum and Kev's relationship and hoped that the holiday would help mend things. Mum and Kev had always got on really well before I became ill; their relationship consisted of boozy family BBQs with lots of banter between the two of them. When I became ill, Mum became much more involved in our lives; she spent most days at our house and discovered how messy, lazy and unreliable Kev can be. She despaired of finding his dirty socks on the lounge floor and a pile of washing up in the sink waiting to be done.

For him, having his mother-in-law around so much was nothing short of a nightmare. He felt he couldn't relax in his own home, because she was critical, snappy, and nothing he ever did was good enough. And I was stuck in the middle, being able to see both perspectives. I tried to explain to Mum that although Kev was far from perfect, he was kind, funny and trying to deal with the worst news imaginable, and I tried to explain to Kev that we couldn't manage without Mum, she was struggling to understand our relationship because it's so different to hers and Dad's and she was dealing with the worst news imaginable too. The holiday was great and, although Mum and Kev got on well, I know they were both making a massive effort. I doubt their relationship will ever be 'good' again, but they seem to have learnt to tolerate each other.

On the last night of our holiday we went out for dinner and I ordered my favourite – seafood risotto. At around 11pm I went to bed feeling a little peculiar, at 2am I woke up and was violently sick, and again at 3am, and 4am, and 5am. By 6am I was suffering from diarrhoea. I felt wretched in the morning; memories of chemo came flooding back. Mum phoned Ward 10 to find out what we needed to do, and was told to call an ambulance and to make sure she told the paramedics about my condition. The ambulance came and I was given a thorough checking over; they were happy that it was 'just' food poisoning. I felt embarrassed at all the fuss, but too weak to argue. We were supposed to leave the chalet by 11am, but I was in no fit state to be moved. The staff at Centre Parcs were very kind and told us to take our time – but ultimately we did have to leave. By about midday my stomach seemed to have settled slightly and there had been no activity for an hour, and so we decided to take the plunge. I was bundled into the car with a sick bowl on my lap and some of the girls' padded bed mats under me. Mum told Kev to drive nice and gently so as not to make me feel worse, but as soon as she'd shut the door, I told him to put his foot down and get me to a bed as soon as possible. The whole experience really shook me; the memories of the chemo haunted me for days afterwards, and the fact that I could suffer everyday illnesses as well as having cancer came as a bit of a shock. Having heard other people's reports of food poisoning, I don't think I had it any worse than anyone else, but I felt that I did. I felt weak and sorry for myself, and that this was the most unfair thing to happen. I have never eaten seafood risotto again.

One of my birthday presents was a voucher for a ride on the London Eye and a Thames lunch cruise. I decided to take my friend Cathy (Kev is scared of heights and refused to go). We had a really special time, staying in the smallest hotel room in the world – well, Cathy had said, "Make it cheap and cheerful," and it certainly was that. I honestly don't think Kev would have fitted in the bathroom.

We spent the first day shopping, before meeting friends for dinner, and then on the second day we did the Thames cruise and treated ourselves to champagne, before using our special tickets to queue jump and take the breath-taking ride on the Eye. Those two days are up there in my special memory bank, as I'm sure they are for Cathy too.

When Kev's mum told us that her friend, who owned a caravan in Weymouth, wanted to offer us her van for a week at a largely discounted price, we jumped at the chance, feeling that we needed to keep making happy memories and fill my last months with happy times. We had a lovely time, but I think Leah summed things up when she exclaimed, "What? Another holiday, Mummy?"

Our lives had been one long holiday, and to be honest it was exhausting trying to maintain that level of fun and excitement. Kev and I realised that we'd need to calm things down if we wanted the girls to grow up well-rounded, with realistic expectations from life. We'd had a very special summer, taken lots of photos and made many happy memories, now it was time to chill out, become more settled for the girls, and accept that maybe I had more time left than I had anticipated.

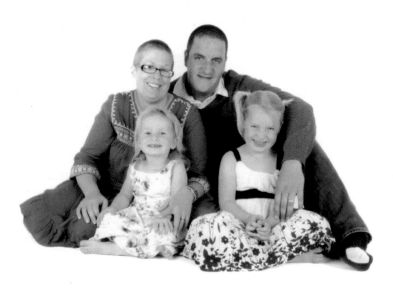

Family studio photo, 2009

10

More medical stuff

After the abuse of the chemotherapy, my veins began to play up whenever the nurses tried to cannulate me for my Herceptin and Zoledronate, and taking blood was becoming an issue too. Although I wasn't keen, the nurses convinced me that a tunnelled central line would be a good move (this is a small catheter placed in the neck or chest, and used to administer medication and fluids and to obtain blood). I knew it had to be done; it was becoming so traumatic for me and the nurses when it took them three or more attempts to get a needle into my arm, but the thought of having a tube sticking out of my chest wasn't hugely appealing.

The procedure was explained to me and I was told that local anaesthetic is all most people need, but if during the operation I felt I needed something stronger, then I was just to let the doctor know. That didn't sound very pleasant … but if it's how most people have it done, then it can't be that bad.

That night I wrote in my diary, 'Well, that was the most hideous thing ever.' The procedure hurt so much, and even though I'd been told to ask for more pain relief, the doctor doing the op just carried on, ignoring my cries of pain and my tears. A kind nurse held my hand, but to be honest that just annoyed me, because if she could see I was in pain, why couldn't the doctor? When it was all over, I had to go for an x-ray to make sure the tube had been inserted into the correct place. I sat in the corridor waiting for my x-ray, thinking about what had happened, experiencing the pain all over again with tears streaming down my face – not one person asked me if I was OK, not even the x-ray staff, or the porter who wheeled me back up to Ward 10. As soon as I saw Mum, my silent tears turned into full-on sobs. Mum and the nurses comforted me until I could pull myself together enough to tell them what had happened. The nurses were horrified and I continued to well up every time I thought about it for the next few days.

The tunnel line meant life was a lot easier and less traumatic when I had to have my treatment, and it also meant that when I had my CT scans and they couldn't cannulate me, I could have the contrast dye through my line. I knew they didn't like doing it that way, because ideally the dye needs to be injected at a higher pressure than the line allows, but it was still an option. Having had two CT scans using my line, I then began to ask if they could use my line without trying to cannulate me first. The first time I asked, the doctor looking after me checked my notes, saw the trouble they'd had in the past and agreed.

When I went for the following scan, I felt unusually relaxed as I waited in the waiting room, because I knew I wouldn't have to go through the trauma of the cannulation. However, the doctor looking after me that day had different ideas – he insisted the contrast needed to go through a vein, because of the pressure issue. I explained that my veins didn't work, but he insisted. Needless-to-say the nurse couldn't cannulate me, and they ended up using my line.

The same thing happened the next time as well. I was so angry and upset; I couldn't seem to make the doctor understand that there was no point in going through the stress of attempted cannulation, only to have to use my line anyway. After my scan I went to PALS (Patient Advice and Liaison Service) and they told me to make my complaint in writing. I received a letter explaining everything I already knew about the contrast dye needing to be administered under pressure, however they agreed that if I telephoned in advance and asked to be put on a 'hot list', they would ensure I was on the list of a doctor qualified in using tunnel lines – and suddenly my doctor's reluctance (due to lack of experience in using tunnel lines) became understandable. Ironically, after my next scan I developed an allergic reaction to contrast dye and have never been able to use it since.

Unfortunately, tunnel lines don't come without their problems. Sometimes they become pressed against something inside and instead of giving up blood, a vacuum would be created. If this happened, I would have to try coughing, waving my arms above my head, and once, even lying down, with the nurse lowering the head of the bed so I was laid with my head lower than my heels in an attempt to shift the tube – sometimes it worked.

Every week, my line had to be bled and flushed through with saline to reduce risk of infection. I watched the district nurse do this so many times and then asked to be taught to do it myself. She was happy because it saved her a job, and this worked well for several weeks. I felt a weird fascination performing the procedure on myself and enjoyed the responsibility. Unfortunately, on one occasion I forgot to do the final flush and a small amount of blood that was left in the tube, dried and caused a blockage. I had to have the line removed. This could be done on Ward 10 with only local anaesthetic, and I was very nervous because of what had happened when it had been inserted, but it was fine. Dr George (Dr Hickish's registrar) did the removal; he said it usually takes from five minutes to half an hour, but in my case it took two hours, because so much scar tissue had formed around the site and it needed to be cut through to release the line.

Having had the line removed, I tried treatment via cannulation again and was disappointed that my veins hadn't recovered enough. I was booked for another tunnel line insertion. This time I insisted on full sedation. The nurses tried to talk me out of it, saying it isn't usually necessary, but I put my foot down. I did feel a bit of a wimp, wondering how these tough guys handled it, but there was no way I was going to risk that level of pain again. I ended up having four lines in total over a period of two years, and each time they tried to persuade me to go without sedation – I didn't once agree.

My final line came out after I was hospitalized with an infection found at the exit site. After two years of walking around with a tube sticking out of my chest, I was thrilled when we discovered my veins had recovered enough to not need a new one.

As women, we become used to doctors prodding and poking our bodies from an early age, with any remaining scrap of dignity being lost at the birth of our children – or so I thought. Another regular appointment I had to attend was for echocardiograms, again, every twelve weeks. This involves sitting on a bed, stripped from the waist up. I find it mortifying having someone, albeit a medical professional, moving my breasts around like lumps of meat. Sometimes they give you a piece of paper sheet to cover yourself, and this sheet invariably falls off or doesn't completely cover you anyway. I find myself trying to preserve my decency with my arms and getting in the sonographer's way. Give me a smear test any day.

11

Supporting my children

Leah was due to start school in September 2009. Before I was diagnosed, I'd looked around a couple of schools and we were pleased that she had been accepted at the local primary school just ten minutes' walk from our house. I decided I needed to talk to someone at the school about my situation and how they would support Leah, so I phoned the school and told the secretary that I had cancer and that my daughter was starting with them in September. She told me I needed to make an appointment with the Family Support Worker. A week later I went to the school, where I was met by a very friendly-looking lady, who showed me through to her office. As we sat down she rested her hand on my arm in a very dramatic fashion and said that before we started she had something to tell me.

"I was diagnosed with breast cancer myself yesterday," she announced.

I was gobsmacked. My initial reaction was to ask what on earth she was doing at work, and she explained that she felt she needed to keep busy. As I walked home, I wondered who had needed the conversation more – me or her. However, I couldn't help but smile at the idea of my baby about to start out on this new journey in her life.

A few weeks later, Kev and I went to a meeting at the school, an introduction for all new parents. There was a girl from Year 6 (ten years old) who did a little talk about being at the school. She was so confident, and I could imagine Leah being like that at her age. Of course, that just made me feel so sad; the idea of her going through her school career without me by her side brought tears to my eyes.

In September, Leah went off happily and has settled in well.

She talks openly about my illness and there have been a couple of occasions where she has become tearful and needed a bit of extra support. Her teachers usually encourage her to make me a card or write me a letter, and that will cheer her up.

The support we have had from the school has been amazing and there has only been one incident that I felt shouldn't have happened. To be honest I would not have been unhappy about it if I hadn't been ill, but considering my prognosis I was furious. Leah came home from school one day having had a supply teacher. I am unsure of the context in which the comment was made, but Leah came home believing that all she needed to do was say a little prayer and I would get better. I was horrified – even the most devout Christians don't believe that prayer can heal terminal illnesses. I spoke to the Head Teacher the next day and explained that I felt it was an irresponsible thing to say – especially given my situation, but that I would have been unhappy about it even if I had been fighting fit, because it just isn't true. The Head Teacher was apologetic and said she'd look into it. I knew that nothing could be done, the comment had been made, but I'm pleased I raised it with the Head so that she was aware and the teacher could be spoken to.

It led to another conversation with Leah about how I am never going to get better. For the first, and only, time she asked me if I was going to die. I swallowed the lump in my throat and explained how everyone dies at some point, most people live to be very old, but sometimes people get ill or are in an accident, which means they die younger. We talked about Uncle Pete and his illness, and I told her that I didn't have any plans to be dying just yet, that the doctors were doing everything they could to keep me well and that the medicine is working well at the moment. I couldn't help feel a little hurt when she said, "Oh, OK, can I have a biscuit now please?" but I was pleased she was able to hear the information and move on so quickly in the way that only children can.

I haven't found it necessary to sit the girls down and make a big announcement about my illness and what the future may hold; I believe that answering any questions they may have, when they have them, is the best way to deal with it. However, we haven't shied away from the subject of death. When Michael Jackson died, we had the funeral on the TV in the background, perhaps many parents would consider it inappropriate viewing for five and three year olds, but when his daughter made a speech it prompted Leah to ask who she was, and then lead onto a conversation about how sad she must feel that her daddy had died. I felt it had been a good lesson to help Leah understand that mummies and daddies can die when their children are still small. So we don't dwell on it, but we are a lot more open about things than we may have been if I were fit and healthy.

Having worked for Bournemouth Adoption Team, preparing children for their move to a new home, I have experience of what is considered best practise in equipping a child for such a major upheaval and emotional trauma. Part of my job was to prepare books for the children about their birth families, because research shows 'It is difficult to grow up as a psychologically healthy adult if one is denied access to one's own history.' – Vera Fahlberg 1991.

Having this knowledge of child psychology, I got to thinking about what I could do for Leah and Megan, about how best to inform them of the things most mums will tell their daughters as they are growing up. I decided to make them a 'Mummy Book' each; I bought two beautiful albums and filled them with my life story. I started with my baby photos, through childhood and adolescence, early adulthood and to when they were born. I included pictures of my best friends, wedding photos and their baby photos. I put small snippets of writing, labelling the photos and talking a bit about myself at the time they were taken. I explained briefly about my diagnosis in a child-friendly way, about how our bodies are made up of building blocks called cells and that my cells are growing too fast and damaging my body. I then put in lots of photos of myself with the respective daughter, from their birth through to now.

It was an overwhelmingly emotional task, but again, something I found very cathartic. I also bought a journal-style notebook each and started writing to each of them about their lives, about my pregnancy with them, their births and early years, telling them the sort of thing I expect they'll want to know when they are expecting their first babies.

I've always been a bit of a hoarder, so the girls both have their own memory boxes, where we have kept all sorts of things, from their first pair of shoes to cinema tickets. I wondered about making 'Mummy memory boxes' so that each of them has special things of mine to remember me by; this is recommended by bereavement experts and I'm sure works for some people, but I felt this was something they may find useful to do for themselves after I'm gone. I've made sure I have two of things they may like to keep. For example I used to have sitting on my pillow a teddy bear that Kev had bought me; I made sure I got another one so that they could have one each. As it turns out, I now have three bears, which is great for times when we are separated (hospital stays or just weekends away); all three of us have a bear to think of each other by. I know this was very valuable, particularly to Megan, when Kev and I went to Los Angeles on holiday and they stayed with my parents for five days. Each night Megan hugged my bear and sent a message to me through him. When I am buried I will have my bear in my coffin and the girls will have theirs to keep.

Another thing that is suggested by bereavement experts is to leave birthday cards behind for your children. Again, I thought about this and felt that it wasn't for me; I wouldn't know when to stop and felt that when I did stop, it would be another loss for them. So, I decided to write a card for special occasions – 13th birthdays, 18th birthdays and wedding days. I felt these were significant events that I needed to mark for them.

I felt that my job really helped me to know what to do for the best in these matters, and am thankful I have the understanding that I do. However some of my knowledge I felt was a mixed blessing. Not long before I finished work, I attended an in-depth training course by a lady called Kate Cairns ('Attachment, Trauma & Resilience', 2002). Her research has further developed the 1969 'Attachment Theory' by John Bowlby, who believed 'that an infant needs to develop a relationship with at least one primary caregiver for social and emotional development to occur normally'.

Kate Cairns explained how a secure attachment in a baby's early years will promote resilience, which is 'the capacity in humans to continue healthy development even through adverse circumstances'. People who are resilient are more likely to recover spontaneously from trauma (emotional as well as physical).

I remembered this and couldn't stop thinking about it, because the girls have a secure attachment to both Kev and me, they have every potential to fully recover from the trauma of losing their mother, especially when their mother has left behind so much information about their immediate history. Of course this is fantastic, and as a mother I feel proud that I will have enabled them to move on and have emotionally healthy lives, but there's part of me, and at the time it was a big part of me, that felt resentful. I hated the fact that they will be fine without me. As a mother I need them to need me and I wasn't prepared to think about them moving on without me. My counsellor helped me come to terms with these feelings and to acknowledge that I have done my best for my girls, and also to be gentle with myself because these feelings are completely understandable.

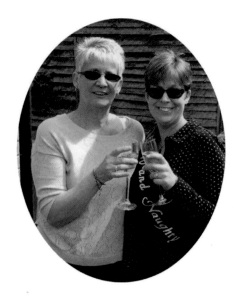

Toasting Nic's 40th birthday

12

Courage and resourcefulness

Here the narrative is taken up by Nikki's mum, Ann Carter ...

'Nic now needed all her courage and resourcefulness as she prepared her girls for a future without her. The photo albums came out and scrapbooking began in earnest. Nic created memory boxes full of treasures from fun times, and scrapbooks full of photos, with a special 'Mummy' book for each of the girls. Having lived with Mummy's cancer for most of their lives, these treasures and memories would help them come to terms with what would happen, enabling them to grow into strong independent women like their mummy.

Nic explains in her 'Mummy' books that no one is to blame for the fact that she has cancer; it is 'just one of those things' ... nobody's fault. She explains in simple terms what cancer does to the body, so the girls will understand what she is going through.

We started video recording, so that they will be able to listen to her voice in the future and see her having fun and messing around with them, like any other mum. Despite her fragile bones, Nic was determined to take part in as many activities with the girls (and her nephews and nieces) as she could; indeed we believe that bouncing on the trampoline with Thom may have been when she sustained a cracked rib. When I suggested to her that maybe she should not have been bouncing, she told me that what was left of her life had to be worth living. She was, of course, so right.

13

'Be careful what you wish for ...'

On Sunday June 21st 2009, Mum, Dannielle, Auntie Cilla, Jan, Charlene, a few others and I entered the Cancer Research UK 'Race for Life' – a five kilometre run, jog, or walk between the Bournemouth and Boscombe piers. I had taken part once before and knew that it was an incredible experience, involving 3,000 women and girls, most wearing pink and many with poignant messages on their backs, stating their reasons for participating.

I prepared for the race by purchasing a tee-shirt bearing the slogan 'I'm a Fighter, not a Victim', but despite my brave declaration, I was concerned about my ability to actually complete the five kilometres, so I arranged for my Uncle Steve to be at the half way point with a wheelchair.

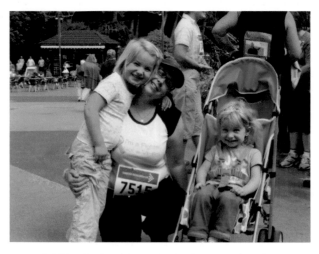

Nikki with the girls, ready for the 'Race for Life'

It was a bright, sunny morning. Kev and the girls, and some other friends cheered us on from the side-lines, and we fell into a slow, but comfortable, pace and enjoyed the walk. Reading the messages on people's backs brought tears to my eyes, but I couldn't stop myself reading them, they were both inspiring and heart-breaking at the same time. I wanted to know what made all these women unite for the same cause.

When we got to the half-way point, I was feeling tired and so put my back-up plan into action. Mum and Cilla took turns pushing me back to Bournemouth. I'm not normally one for being centre of attention, but on this occasion I revelled in the looks of respect I received, and when I decided to get up and walk over the finish line, I knew I was saying, 'Look at me, look at me.' But I didn't care, I was thrilled by the love and support I felt from the supporters and other participants.

As we received our medals, I was approached by a Cancer Research UK (CRUK) press officer, and she asked if I would like to share my story. She explained that a large percentage of sponsor money never gets paid in after the R4L and she was planning to write an appeal to appear in the Bournemouth Echo, encouraging people to pay in their money. Her name was Helen and she wanted to feature someone's story – was I interested? I told her I was and gave her my number.

The next day, I spoke at length to her on the phone. I talked about my diagnosis and how I've been dealing with the changes in my life. I also talked about the girls and the 'Mummy books' I had been making, and we arranged a date for a photographer to come and take a picture of me and the girls. Just before the photographer was due to arrive, Megan was running around naked (as she often did at that age) and I had to blackmail her with sweets, as well as ironing a particular dress that, according to her, was the only one to be worn when meeting the press.

A few days later, I opened the Echo to the headline 'Memories of Me' and a gorgeous photo of me and the girls, headlined 'Terminally ill mum Nikki Hastings is making sure her young girls will never forget her'. The piece talked about my diagnosis, prognosis and how we as a family were dealing with the roller coaster we had been on, including my journal writing.

It felt strange seeing my photo and personal details in print like that, but the few lines at the end, where it said I had shared my story to encourage all those who had taken part in the R4L to return their sponsorship money, made me feel really proud. I felt that if I'd moved one or two people into making their payments, then it had been worth it.

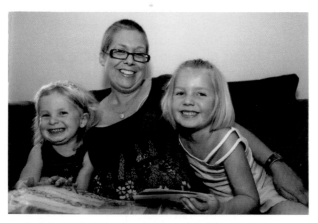

In July 2009, following the Race for Life, this photo was used by Bournemouth echo to thank people for helping Nikki raise £1,000 for CRUK

Later that day, Helen phoned me again. She told me that the Echo journalist, Paula, who had produced her story, had been particularly interested in my comment about my journal. They were wondering how I would feel about having my journal entries printed in the Echo and as an online blog. Helen asked if I would be prepared to meet with Paula to discuss the idea further.

We met, and Paula explained her idea of writing a much bigger story about my situation and putting my journal entries online in a daily blog. She said she would put a link from the blog to a JustGiving page, so people could read my entries and be moved into making a donation to Cancer Research UK. I was immediately interested, I found talking about my illness very therapeutic and this was a way to reach even more people. I talked it through with Mum and Kev. Mum was really reluctant and Kev was really keen. I've always struggled to make decisions on my own – I hate the responsibility of getting it wrong, so to have the two most important people in my life disagreeing over something so big was hard. Mum explained that she felt it would expose me to too many people and make me vulnerable, but she acknowledged that it was my decision and agreed to support whatever I decided. On the next day I phoned Paula and said I wanted to go ahead, so I scanned my diary pages and emailed them over to her.

I had to have more photos taken, this time on my own. Apparently, the best light was in my front porch, so I had to pose against the door frame – I'm sure the neighbours wondered what on earth was going on.

The next day, Mum, Mel and I were booked in for a spa day and overnight stay in a hotel in town.

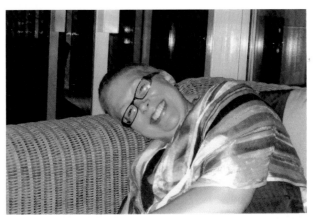

Nikki on a pamper day; the day after her
blog was first printed in the Bournemouth Echo, 2009

I packed my bridesmaid dress and heels to wear to our evening meal, and was gutted when my ankles hurt so much I couldn't wear the shoes, I had to borrow Mel's flip flops and pray that I didn't meet anyone I knew. Being in a hotel on the day that my journal was released to the public may have been a mistake. I nervously opened the paper and seeing my picture and my words in black and white was such a horrible feeling. The headline 'I can't even think about my girls – I don't want to die and leave them' brought a lump to my throat and tears to my eyes. I felt very exposed, and scared that I would get negative feedback. All I wanted to do was cuddle Leah and Megan.

They had also printed a letter I had written to my cancer, something my counsellor suggested I do ...

A letter to my cancer -

'Where did you come from? Why didn't you give me the chance to fight you? It wasn't fair the way you crept up on me and took over my body without me knowing. How did I miss you being there? How did I not know?

What you have done to me is cruel beyond description. You are snatching a young wife and mother in the prime of her life, and for what? My babies are going to have to face life's challenges without me and my husband is going to have to do the same, and support them too on his own, because of your cowardly, evil manipulation of the human body. Surely you could have found someone else? Not that I would wish this on anybody, but why not someone already old or ill or evil? Why me? Why? Why? Why?

I hate you and what you are doing more than I can say, but I won't let it be for nothing. I'm going to make my fight and my death something to be proud of, so that something good can come out of it and so that ultimately I win – not you.'

It all felt too much and I wondered if I'd made a huge mistake.

Getting home on the next day, I felt differently again – there were four letters waiting for me from news agencies, offering me money to tell my story in a national newspaper or women's magazine. Being in my own home made me feel more in control. I decided to give myself time to think about things and see how the Echo blog was received. I set up a Facebook group, 'Nikki's Journal', so that my friends could tell their friends and so on, and in just one month I raised £1,000. I also received overwhelming support, with loving messages from people I'd never met, and such positive feedback from my friends.

The positive reaction prompted my decision to contact the

news agency that had written the most sensitive letter, following the Echo stories. I spoke to a very sympathetic lady, who asked lots of questions about what I had been through over the past few months. She said she'd make some phone calls to see if there was any interest. On the next day she phoned back to say that a popular women's magazine had offered £800 for the story, if I agreed to appear in their Christmas issue with a Christmassy photo shoot included. In the pit of my stomach I was unsure about this. I spoke to Leah to see how she felt about having a pretend Christmas and then felt angry with myself – she's four years old for goodness sake, and of course she's going to feel excited about anything I suggest, especially pretending to have an early Christmas. Mum was even more against this than she had been about the Echo, which was hard for me to deal with, but ultimately I wanted to do it, I wanted the money and I wanted the publicity, and so I convinced myself I was doing it for the right reasons.

A few weeks later the journalist phoned back to read me the story. It was awful, hearing my story told in the first person, but using words and expressions that I would never have used. I didn't have the opportunity to read the piece in my own time; she read it through once and I had to agree there and then – I didn't feel I had a choice, I had come this far and I had to agree. This was in the September; I was told that the magazine would be in touch at the end of October to arrange the photo shoot. The photographer phoned one evening to discuss what they needed and to arrange a convenient time. We discussed Christmas trees, presents, the girls in fairy costumes (why fairies I don't know), etc. He then told me that they needed some old photos – one from before my illness and one of me with no hair. He then said, "Don't worry if you kept your hair throughout, we'll just shave it off for the photo." I didn't know how to react; I gave a nervous chuckle and ended the conversation, agreeing to see him on the arranged date.

I put the phone down and burst into tears – I really wasn't sure if he'd been serious or if it had been a terrible joke. If I had kept my hair, was he implying I hadn't suffered enough? If I had lost it and re-grown it, did he really think I'd want to cut it again?

It really hit me then that all they were interested in was sensationalising the story. How dishonest to their readers – I felt totally exploited.

On the next day I phoned the news agency and said I wanted to pull out. I was surprised by their understanding at losing a commission. The day after, I received a bouquet of flowers and a 'sorry' card. I was relieved the whole thing was over; I had felt unsure for a while, but had been bowled along by the process.

I decided to keep the material and write a book, my story, straight from the horse's mouth.

14

The media effect

The media is such a huge part of everyday life ... it's impossible to escape it. Jade Goody (Big Brother contestant) was diagnosed with cervical cancer in August 2008, two months before my own diagnosis. In February 2009 it was announced that her cancer had spread and was now terminal. I watched the portrayal of her illness played out through the TV and newspapers, and it was really tough. Many people criticised her for being so public, and perhaps I would have done too had I not been in such a similar situation. I understood her need to share her experiences with people. I found it so therapeutic just talking and talking to anyone who would listen – she just had a bigger audience.

When it came to her last days of life, I was terrified, seeing the headlines telling of her loss of sight, the pain she was in, and that she had been hallucinating. Before that I hadn't considered the facts of death ... just that I was going to die. I hadn't thought about the pain or any other related conditions, and seeing what she was going through so graphically, really affected me. I didn't want to be in pain, I didn't want to lose my sight or not know who I was. I didn't want to go through what Jade was going through and didn't want to hear all about it.

Patrick Swayze was another celebrity who went through his cancer at the same time as me. He was less in the public eye than Jade, but seeing headlines reporting him working through chemo and refusing pain relief because he didn't want it affecting his mind, I found quite upsetting. It made me feel inadequate, and that I was being a wimp by not being able to work and relying so heavily on pain killers.

It took a while for me to get my head around the fact that everyone is different and everyone's cancer is different. There was a newspaper story reporting a new treatment that Patrick had received, called 'Cyberknife Radiosurgery'. The article prompted Mum to email a Harley Street doctor to enquire whether this treatment would be suitable for me. It was a difficult time waiting for the reply; it's hard not to get your hopes up when you think all options have been considered and then something new comes up. Needless-to-say, the response was negative – Cyberknife surgery is used to accurately target small tumours more directly than traditional radiotherapy. In my case I have spots of cancer cells throughout my body, so the treatment would be inappropriate. It was hard not to feel disappointed, even though I had known it was a long shot.

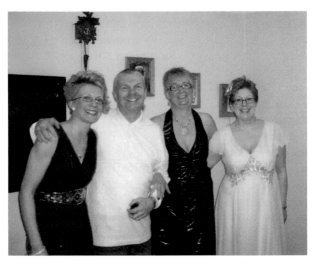

Nikki with Mel and her mum and dad
going to the Pink Ball, March 2011

In December 2011 the BBC ran a big story about how 40% of cancers are due to lifestyle choices and could be prevented by not drinking, smoking or eating the wrong things. Stories like that are really hard to hear. It felt as if the media were blaming me for my situation and I could have prevented my condition by living my life differently. So often there are news reports about how different foods can cause or help prevent cancer – it can be mind boggling, especially when you get conflicting advice. I have learnt to take it all with a pinch of salt. The media can be very useful in informing our choices, but we have to be sensible about it ... we have to enjoy our lives. We all know stories of someone's granddad who smoked twenty cigarettes a day since he was fifteen and is still fine, but we also know that smoking can cause cancer – so we have to make informed choices and hope for the best.

I will never know if my lifestyle contributed towards my illness, so I can't keep wishing I'd done things differently. My tastes have changed greatly since being diagnosed – I feel nauseous so often that I really do have to eat whatever I fancy. I couldn't live on a diet of only raw fruit and vegetables, even if I wanted to, and I listen to my body, which often craves cheese, despite knowing that many people believe dairy products can cause and promote the growth of breast cancer.

15

A blast from the past

When my first marriage broke up, my ex and I agreed that we would stay friends, but after a year or so we had little in common and went our separate ways. I was upset when one Christmas I popped round to our old flat with a card for him, to discover he had sold up and moved on. There were sightings of him by others, but in over ten years I never once bumped into him, even though he had remained in the local area. After my diagnosis, I wondered several times if I should contact him, I was already back in touch with the rest of our friendship group from back in those days. It felt wrong that Matt wasn't part of it, and it felt wrong that he didn't know about me. I talked it through with Mum and Kev, who both felt it was best to leave it, there was no point in raking up the past – but I couldn't stop thinking about him and knowing that if the situation were reversed, I would want to know about him.

I decided I would write to his mum – after all I knew nothing about Matt's new situation, he may have an insecure partner who wouldn't cope with me turning up out of the blue, this being my main concern. I explained that I didn't want anything from Matt, just that I felt he should know, and I asked his mum to make the decision for me and to let me know if she decided to tell him or not. I didn't hear anything from her and took that as a sign to forget about it.

Once my blog was in the Echo I thought about him again and wondered if he'd seen my story. I tracked him down through 192.com and one evening when Kev was out, I took the plunge and called him. A woman answered the phone and said he was out. I said that I was Nikki and knew him from way back, and she immediately asked if I had been married to him. It was really weird talking to her; I was almost disappointed that she sounded lovely. I asked if they'd heard my news – they hadn't, and when I told her, she was very sympathetic. We chatted for a while; she told me about their daughter and I told her about Kev and the girls. She also mentioned that they had been talking about me recently, because my name was still on one of Matt's insurance policies. She said she would get him to call me back.

I was pretty shaken when I put the phone down. It was good to hear that he was happy and settled, but I felt very emotional. I phoned Cathy and couldn't help my tears. She came straight over with wine and chocolate.

On the next day, I thought about the insurance policy; I did remember there being an issue with a policy, because it was an endowment that we couldn't change the names on, or something similar. I decided to speak to a financial advisor before I spoke to Matt, to find out where I stood. He explained that if my name is on the policy and the payments are all up to date, then it would be payable on my death and the money would go to my estate – which Kev and the girls would inherit, meaning that Matt would have paid into this policy for all these years and could lose it all.

I had a horrible feeling in my stomach; I couldn't believe that after all these years of not being in touch, the first thing we needed to deal with was negotiating a financial matter.

Matt phoned later that day; we chatted for a while – their daughter is also called Megan. That freaked me out, especially because when we were together we hadn't got as far as discussing children, so didn't have any baby names planned – how weird that if we had stayed together and had children, Megan would possibly have been the name we'd have picked.

Then we got onto the insurance policy; he told me that it had critical illness cover so we could claim on it now. He suggested he would work out how much he'd paid into it, take that out and then split the difference 50/50 with me. I felt impressed by his generosity, angry that he got to benefit from my illness, and then grateful that he had kept up the payments so that we both get a nice, unexpected windfall.

We met up for me to sign the necessary forms. I was shocked at how he hadn't changed at all; we chatted about our families and I said 'hello' to his wife, who was sat in the car. I realised then that the stuff I really wanted to say – acknowledging that we were once very special to each other, telling him I forgive him for our marriage breakdown, because I'm happy, and I'm pleased he's happy – that was going to always remain unsaid – we've moved on. That was the last time I saw or spoke to him, but I will always be very grateful for the money that was deposited into my bank account in time to make my second 'final Christmas' another very special time, and allowing me to clear the last of our debts in the debt management plan.

16

It's not all bad

Despite the devastation that cancer causes, it is undeniable that opportunities arise which probably never would have done without a cancer (or other critical illness) diagnosis.

The Echo journalist, Paula, who wrote the stories relating to my blog, happened to know a lady who worked for Bournemouth Tourism, and that lady asked Paula to ask me if I wanted a family VIP ticket to the second Bournemouth Air Festival. Did I ever?! Kev, the girls and I were treated to a fantastic day, including a three course lunch, afternoon tea, free flowing wine and seats in prime position to see the best of the flying displays and hear the commentary – all because a friend of someone I knew was moved by my story.

My brother-in-law Morgan played rugby, and on hearing my news his club secretary suggested a charity day to raise money for the cancer charity of my choice. They called the day 'Balls to Breast Cancer'. Although I got involved with collecting some raffle prizes, most of the day was organised by the club members. We kicked off with a curry lunch, then the lads played rugby in pink shirts (all making donations for the privilege), and then more food, before the grand auction and raffle. We raised £5,000 that day, and I was moved to tears when they announced that they wanted us to have £3,000 of it to take the girls to Disneyland, Paris. The rest of the money was split between The Willow Foundation and Macmillan.

The holiday was so special; it really was a once in a lifetime trip, we could afford to do all the extras – shows, treat the girls to souvenirs and lunch with the Princesses – and all because someone who knew someone I know was moved by my story.

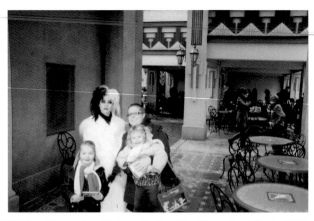

Nikki and her girls with Cruella Deville, Disneyland Paris, 2010

I wanted a donation from the money raised through Balls to Breast Cancer to go to The Willow Foundation, because when I was first diagnosed they paid for us to have a two day visit to Legoland and a night in a hotel. They are an organisation that provides special treats for young people (under 40 years) who have a serious illness. That day out for us meant a lot, because Legoland was the last place we'd been on a family day out before I was ill (on that occasion using Tesco Clubcard vouchers to pay for a one day visit). Our special day, courtesy of The Willow Foundation, felt like we were putting two fingers up to my cancer by doing it bigger and better, despite my illness.

I struggled with these opportunities, because it felt wrong to be enjoying ourselves so much – as if we were saying 'Life is better now I have cancer' – which on the surface, in some ways it was – but I'd have given it all up in a flash to have my health back. At least this way I was enjoying the time I had left, and I was creating happy memories for Kev, Leah and Megan.

Taking advantage of my illness, or 'playing the cancer card' as some people term it, didn't come naturally to me; I'd been brought up to 'put up and carry on'. It soon became clear that there were 'perks' that I could take advantage of. Being on welfare benefits went against everything I believed in, but when I thought about it rationally, I realised I had to apply. I couldn't work, even if I felt well enough, which I didn't – I had too many appointments to manage, so when the hospital social worker asked me to describe how I felt on my worst days so she could make my claim, I didn't hold back.

Having a Blue Badge so that I could park in disabled spaces or on double yellow lines when I needed to, felt really wrong. A friend told me to only use it if it meant going somewhere that I would have otherwise avoided due to concern about parking. I found her advice helpful and so don't use it to use a disabled space that's closer to the Tesco door, but I do use it when I get home with my shopping to park on the double yellow lines outside my house whilst I unpack my shopping, have a cup of tea and put my feet up before finding a parking space. I was aware of the false limp I developed when I first used it, but I'm pleased to say that soon disappeared as my confidence grew.

On another occasion, Cathy took me out for dinner as a birthday treat. I went to go to the toilet and when I discovered they were down a flight of very steep stairs I decided that as I was wearing high heels and my hip was niggling a bit, I would be safer and more comfortable using the disabled toilet on the ground floor. The sign on the door said to ask a member of staff for the key, but when I did so, the waitress looked me up and down and said, "Do you really need to use the disabled toilet." I felt my cheeks burn as the table of people next to us all stopped eating and stared at me. I told her that I had cancer in my bones and that my hip was painful, so yes please, could I have the key. She grudgingly handed it over; I finished my meal, went home and emailed the manager suggesting diversity training for his staff, and I received a voucher for a free meal by way of apology.

The whole 'disability' issue can be very contentious – one night at a concert at the BIC, I went to use the disabled toilet. There was a lady in front of me using walking sticks, and the toilet was engaged when I joined the queue. When the door opened two giggly young women came out and the lady with the sticks had a real go at them for using the disabled toilet when there was 'clearly nothing wrong with them'. She then looked at me, looked at my head scarf and said "Don't worry, I'm not talking about you." It struck me then that people consider disability to be something they can see; if it's not visible there's nothing wrong. I'm registered disabled, I receive Disability Living Allowance and cancer is covered by the Disability Discrimination Act – but 80% of the time I look fine. I worry constantly that one day someone is going to accuse me of abusing the system, and I hope that if it happens I'm strong enough to explain why I'm registered disabled, rather than bursting into tears, which I suspect is the reaction that will come most naturally.

17

A cold caller

About three months after The Race for Life, one Sunday tea time I answered the phone to a young chap from Cancer Research UK. The conversation went something like this –

Him – "Good evening Mrs Hastings, and how are you today?"

Me – "I'm fine thank you. Is this going to take long, because I'm just about to sit down to dinner?"

Him – "Don't worry, this won't take long and I'm not asking for money. I wanted to congratulate you on taking part in this year's Race for Life; can I ask what made you sign up for it?"

Me – "Because I have cancer myself."

Him – "Oh, that's brilliant."

Me – "I can assure you it isn't."

Him – "No, no, I'm sure, I sometimes wonder who it's hardest for, those with cancer themselves or those watching a loved one suffer. As one in three of us are now affected by cancer it is something that should be close to us all."

Me – "As I'm sure it is."

Him – "So, do you think you would like to do a bit more to help us? By donating just £10 a month to Cancer Research UK you could make such a difference to our work."

Me – "I thought you weren't phoning to ask for money? ... anyway, due to my illness I'm not really in a position to make a long term financial commitment, I'm afraid."

Him – "I understand that, perhaps just £5 a month then?"

Me – "As well as personal donations in the past, I have already done quite a lot of fundraising for CRUK, not only did myself and several family members do the Race for

Life, my Dad raised over £1,000 doing the ten kilometre run and I have an online blog with a link to a JustGiving page, which has raised over £1,000 for CRUK. I'm happy with the amount I have donated and raised and, as I say, I'm not in a position to make a regular financial commitment."

Him – "That really is fantastic, so perhaps just £3 a month, Mrs Hastings?"

Me – "Goodbye."

I was shocked and angry; did he really say it was brilliant I had cancer? I'm sure he didn't actually mean it was brilliant I had cancer, but that is what he said; he also asked me to think about who suffers most – patients or their loved ones. Did he really want to know what myself and my family have been through, and continue to go through? All evening I played the conversation over and over in my head. Initially it made me feel that I wouldn't donate again and then it worried me that these insensitive call centre staff would put other people off donating, which is something I'd hate to happen as Cancer Research UK do such necessary work. They just need people with more empathy and sensitivity in their call centres.

Kev suggested I speak to Paula, the Echo journalist, about my 'chugging' (Charity Mugging) experience. She passed my comments on to Helen Johnstone, CRUK Press Officer, and asked if they could do a story with an official apology. The angle of the story would be to encourage people to continue donating, despite these insensitive phone calls. I felt excited to be part of something so positive.

The story really put the cat among the pigeons – it described the call, included a public apology with CRUK Head of Donor Development, stating that they were looking into how their call centres work and taking steps to ensure this doesn't happen again, and finished with my quote – "I've had an apology and now want to encourage people to continue to support CRUK and the important work they do."

It was front page of the Echo, and then because the Echo is part of a syndicate, the story was picked up by some of the national newspapers. None of them contacted me; they lifted photos from my JustGiving page and interpreted the story in their own way. It didn't feel so positive at that point, and because the newspapers are now online, their readers have the opportunity to comment on stories. My story received lots of positive comments, supporting me and reporting similar experiences, but also negative comments, criticising me for being so ungrateful in slagging off a charity I have benefited from, many telling me I had misunderstood the use of the word 'brilliant', and another commenting on how I'm happy to raise money by persuading others to hand over their cash and maybe I should put my hand in my own pocket. I felt very vulnerable and hurt that these people didn't understand what I was saying; I wasn't criticising CRUK, just the approach of some of their call centre staff, I encouraged people to keep supporting CRUK and whether I donate personally or not is my business, no one else's – just as it is for everyone.

On the next day Helen Johnstone phoned, because she thought I'd be interested to know that all the senior people at CRUK were aware of what happened and were seriously looking at their use of call centres in their fundraising campaigns. I felt so proud that I managed to achieve that – and whether they've been good to their word, or just scratched my name off all their databases, I don't know, but I've never had a call like that since, even though I have participated in further Race for Life events.

18

Bad scan results

In January 2010 I had a routine CT scan. For some reason I felt uneasy about it; for the first time in the nine months since my chemotherapy ended, I was feeling well, active, and we were having fun as a family. I was worried that it had all got too good to last. I felt despair at myself and the way my mind was working. Previously, just before a scan I would develop aches and pains that worried me sick, this time I was worried because I felt too well.

I had the scan and decided we needed to book the trip to Disneyland, Paris, that the Balls to Breast Cancer money was paying for. Despite the snow that had hit the UK with a vengeance and had caused the cancellation of the Eurostar on a couple of occasions during the week before, I knew we had to go before I got my scan results. I booked the holiday on the Thursday evening, to go the following Wednesday for five days and come back two days before my scan results were due. It all felt very impulsive and exciting, and even though it was very cold, the holiday was magical.

Looking back now on my childhood, I don't think we had much spare money when we were growing up. I would never have known at the time; we were always kept busy and did fun things, but it was walks in the New Forest, Poole Park or Mudeford Quay, and our summer holidays were spent swapping homes with cousins – I would go and stay with Clare whilst her brother David stayed at our house, then a few weeks later Clare would come to us and Matt would go there. Uncle Steve has four sons and there was lots of house swapping that went on with them. We would also have maybe one big day trip; Windsor Safari Park, the Natural History Museum, HMS Victory, Bristol Zoo for example.

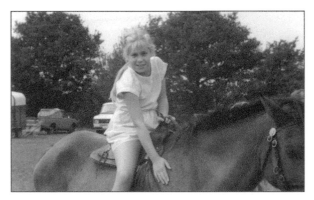

Nikki aged approximately 12

We went away on my first family holiday when I was eight years old, we rented a cottage in Cornwall and drove there in our first family car; a Cortina; a company car for dad. My memories of that holiday were that the cottage had an open staircase and Matt was too scared to go up or down on his own, in case he fell through the gaps. Mel and I played offices or shops on those stairs, sitting on one step with our legs through the gap, using the step above as a desk or till.

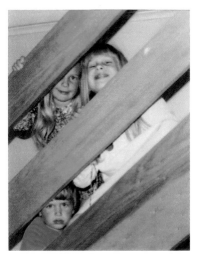

Nikki, Mel and Matt playing on the stairs

Over the years we went on other cottage holidays and then developed a love of camping, even venturing as far as France with Key Camp. I was fourteen years old before I went on an aeroplane. Being able to take Leah and Megan on such a special holiday at such a young age felt like a real privilege.

I wasn't surprised when at my oncology appointment Dr Hickish told me that, although the cancer in my liver and bones was stable, there was also some bad news – my lymph nodes were enlarged, so I needed more chemotherapy. He told me about a new drug that had recently become available, called T-DM1, short for Trastuzumab emtansine (Herceptin is the trade name for the drug Trastuzumab). At the time it was a very new drug, but early reports were promising. The only way I could have T-DM1 was to take part in a trial called the EMILIA trial, a comparative trial between T-DM1 and Capecitabine and Lapatinib together.

I went home with a bundle of information and five days to make my decision. Kev's reaction to the news was very different to mine; he focussed on what Dr Hickish had said about my liver and bones, seeming to me to have completely ignored the bad news, whereas I felt absolutely devastated, terrified of more chemo, and couldn't even think about the rest of my cancer being stable – to me it felt like the beginning of the end. I understood that Kev was trying to protect himself (and probably me too) from the fear of what lies ahead, but I felt his attitude belittled the way I was feeling. He made me think that I was over-reacting and was being silly for being so upset. I remember telling him how insensitive I thought he was, and feeling surprised that he admitted he was wrong.

There was so much going around in my head. I looked on the internet and found reports from women who had been on Lapatinib & Capecitabine for two to three years. The side effects were quite similar to the other chemo drugs I'd been on, but with no hair loss, and the nausea and vomiting were described as 'mild'. I was able to learn that T-DM1 is made up of chemotherapy drugs that had been developed over twenty years ago, but had not been used because of being highly toxic; however, the new combination that is called T-DM1 allows the toxic drug to travel to the cancer cells and work only on them. It was harder to find information about side effects, and I later discovered this was because it was still very early days in the trial and so few had been reported. The difference between the trial and my previous chemo was that I'd be on these drugs indefinitely, for as long as they continued to work – or until I could no longer tolerate the side effects.

The decision process involved other people; I needed to know that Mum could be around for me on a more long term basis – her work had asked her to make a decision about whether she was returning or not (she was at the time still on unpaid compassionate leave, but they needed to know what she wanted to do long term). She felt that she couldn't go back to work, because she wanted to be with me and the girls. She had built up such a close relationship with the girls and she didn't want to leave them now. She also wanted to be there to help me and spend quality time with me. She made the decision to leave work, and Dad supported that decision. I was also hugely relieved to hear that my wonderful Uncle Steve, who had already acted as my own personal taxi service since this all began, was happy to commit to driving me to and from the hospital whenever I needed. It was so good to have such a fantastic support network.

The following week, at my next hospital appointment I met the nurse consultant who would be organising the trial. I told her I was happy to go ahead and she put the wheels in motion. I needed to have lots of scans to ensure I was fit enough to undertake the trial … so another CT scan, an MRI, and a bone scan which involved an injection of radioactive dye and therefore 24 hours of quarantine from the girls.

A week later I had my pre-chemo, which involved blood tests, urine samples, an ECG and a full physical examination, which together with the results of the previous week's scans, meant they were able to decide that I was fit enough to undergo the trial. I was also told that I would be on the T-DM1 arm of the trial. I felt pleased about this, because although Dr Hickish hadn't said it outright, I felt sure that he'd implied this was the one he wanted me on. To say that it felt like the end of my life as

I knew it, seems very melodramatic, but to be facing a future of continuous treatment, with three weekly infusions for the rest of my life was very daunting.

On the next day I went in for my treatment. The first dose had to be infused over 60 minutes, and as long as I had no adverse effects, all future doses could be given over 30 minutes. My nurse told me that I was one of only 580 people worldwide to be taking T-DM1; that made things feel very scary ... I really was a guinea pig.

However, it all went fine; in fact it was a huge anti-climax. When I had chemo before, I had returned home with a long list of dos and don'ts, who to call in an emergency, what not to eat, etc. This time it was all very low key, with no special instructions and nothing to expect.

The following couple of days I felt tired and nauseous, but the nausea was easy to control with tablets, and I slept a lot. The full reaction to the treatment hit me like a ton of bricks exactly a week later.

19

An extreme reaction

Exactly a week after the first dose of my new treatment, Kev and I had a falling out. I had asked him to help out more in the mornings, and on the very next day he grumbled when I didn't feel up to getting up. Mum happened to phone at precisely the wrong moment, because I must have sounded upset and she asked why. Kev heard me telling her that he'd grumbled about having to get the girls ready on his own, and he lost the plot. He went absolutely mad at me for 'telling tales' on him. He got the girls ready, stormed out of the house with them, dropping Leah at school and taking Megan to his mum's. I did something I thought I would never do and involved his mum. I was worried about him and didn't know how to help him. I told my mother-in -law that Kev was angry, explaining, "He's bottling things up and he can't keep this up any longer." I told her that he needed someone to talk to.

Whilst he was at his mum's, my mum came round to see me. After crying and sleeping on her lap, I started to think and talk about the things that made me angry – the way Kev seemed to be in denial, the way he didn't take responsibility for things around the house, the way he went out in the evenings so much … then the post arrived and in it was a parking ticket from outside Kev's friend's house. At that point I was ready to leave him.

When he came home from his mum's we had a tearful heart -to-heart, with lots of crying, shouting and eventually talking. That night I was absolutely drained – my eyes felt gritty where I'd been crying so much, my mind and body were exhausted. Kev put the girls to bed and I told him that as I was going to bed, I didn't mind if he went out.

Of course, once he'd gone I didn't want to be alone any

more. I had the phone in my hand, but I couldn't ring Mum because she'd be angry at Kev for going out, I didn't want to call Mel because Thom was poorly so she needed to be with him, and although I knew Cathy would drop everything and come over, I didn't want that either, because I knew what I really needed to do was sleep. I cried some more and started to think how life would be so much easier if I wasn't here. Feeling like this and living like this just felt so miserable. I was causing Kev so much heartache, and the same for Mum and Dad, and the rest of my family. I didn't want the girls to remember me always crying. It would be better all-round if I ended it.

Those thoughts freaked me out … was I really thinking about killing myself? I didn't know, but I knew I couldn't tell anyone close to me that I was feeling this way. I looked up the number for the Samaritans. I dialled the number several times before I let it ring. It felt so silly to be ringing them. I wasn't serious about ending it … was I?

When the lady answered the phone, I just started crying and repeated over and over how it would be easier for everyone if I was dead. She asked me why I felt like that, so I told her about my cancer, and I told her I was going to die soon anyway and living like this was just agony. To my surprise her response was, "Oh my dear, I just don't know what to say, I'm so sorry. I don't know what to say." I think the ridiculousness of the situation hit me then. I'd managed to render a Samaritan speechless – she deals with seriously screwed-up people every day and didn't know what to say to me. I told her I felt a bit better for talking to her, and she replied, "I'm pleased to have been of some help, goodbye." I think I even laughed as I put the phone down.

The next day was no better – I couldn't stop crying, and I felt so tired. I felt that I'd had enough and couldn't fight any more. I wanted to be on my own and begged Mum and Kev to let me book myself into a hotel. I didn't want anyone; I just wanted to lie in bed and cry – on my own.

Dr Mitchell (my GP) telephoned to see how I'd got on with my new treatment, and when he heard the state I was in he came straight round. He listened and talked, and prescribed Diazepam, to work as an 'emotional cosh'. He explained that the drugs wouldn't make things better, but they'd help numb the pain. Mum told him how I'd been begging to be on my own, and he suggested talking to my palliative care nurse about a hospice place, so Mum telephoned Linda, who told her that there was nowhere available at such short notice. That made me cry because I felt so angry – how can things like this be planned; surely there should be a service to support people in this sort of situation?

I remember lying on my bed, crying into and punching the pillow in anger and frustration. All I wanted was to go somewhere to be on my own – was that really too much to ask?

Mum suggested I go and stay with her and Dad, and the next couple of days were spent in their spare bed, crying, sleeping and being cuddled. On the third day, I woke up feeling a bit brighter. I commented to Mum that I really fancied a massage and what a shame you couldn't get someone to come to your house to do it. Of course that gave Mum something to do, and she went online and make several enquiries, telling people about my condition, my situation and how I didn't want to leave the house. Listening to her negotiations made me feel very panicky – it was too much hassle. I could feel my chest tighten and my breathing becoming shallow as I had my first panic attack.

Mum did manage to find a lady who would come to the house to do a hot stone massage, and a couple of days later I met Stacey. Since that day, Stacey has come to my home to massage me every six weeks or so. I feel it is part of my treatment, it certainly helps me to relax, and who knows what other benefits it provides?

My anger towards Kev began to ease, until I discovered he had another parking ticket. I worried so much about how he was going to manage when he found himself on his own. When we'd been arguing, I told him that I 'carried him'. He was offended and accused me of being unfair. I couldn't understand how he couldn't see that I did everything at home; from making sure we all had clean clothes to wear and food to eat, to managing the finances, paying the bills and finding the extra for his parking tickets. He went out to work full time and I did everything else. I realised it was as much my fault as his, because in the past I had happily done it all. I loved the role of home maker and organiser, and so it suited us both. The problem arose when I became ill – he should have taken over some (if not all) of the household chores and he hadn't.

I knew how much he was struggling with the way our lives had changed, so I didn't force the issue. I really hoped a break from each other was what we both needed to find our feet, however it didn't help when Kev happily announced how easy it was to get the girls ready in the morning and how he had plenty of time to do everything – I'm sure now, that he was just trying to reassure me that they were coping without me, but at the time I felt he was gloating and implying I made a fuss over nothing. It got to the point where I didn't have the energy to feel angry anymore, I just felt so sad.

Mum suggested that I was possibly having some sort of emotional breakdown. That sounded so dramatic, but I suppose she was probably right. I was totally drained, I couldn't pretend that everything was OK anymore, whenever I tried to think about doing anything I became panicky and had several panic attacks, and even the smallest, simplest tasks exhausted me.

A few weeks prior to the start of my new treatment, my girlfriends from university and I had booked tickets to see *Priscilla, Queen of the Desert* in London. We had all been so excited about it, but I was so low I couldn't even think about going. Rhea, Jo, Laura and Lou were very understanding, but they wouldn't let me pull out completely, all saying, "See how you feel on the day."

In the days leading up to the trip, Mum spoke to Uncle Steve and they devised a plan. They knew there was no way I'd even consider going on the train on my own (as had been the plan), so they decided they'd take me in Steve's car, see me to the theatre door, go shopping and then meet me and the girls afterwards. I was still very nervous and panicky about it – I did really want to go, but I didn't want to embarrass myself and everyone else by having a panic attack. Mum and Kev convinced me that it would be good for me to go, see my friends and have a fun day – all in the safety of knowing Mum was close by.

I felt like a baby, but I knew that Mum being there was the only way I would be able to do it. We drove up in plenty of time, and as we approached central London I began to feel panicky. Mum calmed me down, we parked the car, and then went for some lunch. When I met the girls I was overcome with emotion – I cried and cried. I hadn't thought I would make it and yet here we all were. I really didn't think I was going to get through the theatre door and felt like such a drama queen for making all that fuss – but I really couldn't help it. Lots of cuddles and deep breathing helped me to pull myself together. I felt so scared that these silly attacks were going to start affecting what I did and where I went.

The show was spectacular. I had never seen anything like it; the costumes were so over-the-top, there were hilarious one-liners throughout, and the leading men (including Jason Donovan) received standing ovations. I felt so alive and was able to forget about everything for a couple of hours.

After the show Mum and Uncle Steve were waiting outside the theatre for us, they'd had a lovely afternoon, meeting my cousin for coffee and wandering around Covent Garden. My friends and I had booked a table at Pizza Express, around the corner. We asked Mum and Steve to join us, but not wanting to cramp our style, they went to the restaurant next door – close enough if I needed them, which I'm pleased to say I didn't. The day was such a great achievement, although the past week had been a nightmare. Perhaps I was coming through the other side.

Kev and the girls were desperate to have me home; it broke my heart every time I saw them and the girls cried for me to go with them each time they left. The problem was I had become comfortable at Mum and Dad's, spending my time lounging around reading, watching DVDs and generally being looked after. The thought of going home terrified me – I would have to take responsibility again, the panic attacks were a real concern and I didn't want the girls to see me crying all the time. But I still wanted to be with them and felt that living like this wasn't doing them any good.

Linda, my palliative care nurse, visited and was visibly

shocked at the state I was in. She asked me to call Dr Mitchell out again and said that perhaps the Psychiatric Team needed to become involved in my case.

Dr Mitchell visited and said that he wanted my oncologists to consider whether my reaction had been a direct result of the new treatment (a side effect), and if they agreed, suggest what could be done, as I couldn't go through this every three weeks. He also decided to change my anti-depressants to a higher level drug and referred me to the consultant at the local Palliative Care Unit (where they take a more holistic approach to care). Dr Mitchell warned Kev that I had to be weaned off the anti-depressants I was taking before I could start the new ones, and things were likely to get worse before they got better. I couldn't help thinking, 'How is it possible for things to get worse?'

20

A miracle drug?

Thankfully things didn't get any worse, but it took a while for things to get better. Whilst I was being weaned off my old antidepressants, I was using the Diazepam more, which did help with the feelings of despair.

To start with I had an appointment with Dr Pugh, Palliative Medicine Consultant at the Palliative Care Unit, a team who work closely with medical and nursing teams to advise on the provision of good symptom control and psychological, social and spiritual support. She listened to me cry for an hour and a half. In that time I managed to establish that I wasn't ready to die, but that I couldn't continue to live the way I had been. Dr Pugh suggested I started attending the Macmillan Day Centre within the Palliative Care Unit, where I would be able to completely rest, read, do pottery, art classes and, more importantly, spend time with people in the same situation as me.

At my next pre-chemo appointment, I discussed with Dr Hickish the suggestion Dr Mitchell had made about my depression being a reaction to the new chemo. Dr Hickish said it was a definite possibility, but that I'd need to have more to be sure. He felt it was more likely to be a reaction to everything that had happened over the previous year and that it had finally caught up with me. I agreed that he could be right, although I preferred Dr Mitchell's suggestion, because that way it wasn't down to me to sort out.

I had my next dose and, as before, felt tired and sick for the next few days. Then a few days later I had another panic attack (the first in over a week). Megan had a tantrum about something totally normal for a two and a half year old and I just couldn't deal with it. Then a few days later, after we'd had some friends around the previous evening, our upstairs neighbour, Mary, left us a note saying, "Sounds like you guys had fun last night! Just to let you know I'm doing some decorating over the next few days so may be a bit noisy."

I saw red. I started to bang on her door. Kev came out to see what the noise was about and I handed him the note. I saw from his face that he was confused. Thankfully, Mary was out, so I went back into our flat with Kev, ranting about how selfish she was, and how could she make sarcastic little comments and then warn us that she was going to make noise … it must just be to get back at us.

Kev was looking really confused at that point. "I really think she's being genuine in asking if we'd had a good time last night and is just letting us know that she's going to be decorating."

I burst into tears, realising Kev was probably right. I felt mortified that I'd flown off the handle and so thankful that Mary had been out. I couldn't believe I'd got it so wrong and felt scared by the strength of my feelings – I had been so angry.

It happened again a few days later when I thought someone had queue jumped me in a shop. Fortunately, Kev was with me and held me back when he saw that I was about to shout at someone who had taken her turn by merging into the queue I was stood in. I was able to release my anger by ranting at the ridiculous queuing system, but I felt shaken up and afraid that had I been on my own I would have shouted at an innocent person – who may well have turned round and punched me on the nose.

Now, I've always been able to stand up for myself and have even been known to get a bit stroppy at times, but these feelings of pure rage were very out of character and really scared me. I struggled through the next week, experiencing severe mood swings and episodes of irrationality – imagine the worst PMS possible and it going on for at least ten days.

The crunch came when Kev and I had another row. I'd taken Leah to her swimming lesson and asked Kev to peg the washing out whilst I was gone. When I got back, the washing was still in the machine. I went mad, screaming at him for being so unreliable and yelling, "I can't trust you to do anything." I wouldn't listen to him when he tried to explain that his mum had phoned and so he'd been speaking to her for most of the time I'd been gone. Eventually, he walked out, angry and frustrated.

Later that day, Mum and I took the girls to a fete at the school. Kev phoned me whilst we were there and I remember walking round the school hall, with tears streaming down my face, trying not to raise my voice as Kev told me how unreasonable I was and how he couldn't deal with it any more. I told him I would have to stop the treatment, to which he shouted, "And then you'll bloody die." I felt that I had no option; I was convinced it was the drugs turning me into a monster for ten days out of twenty one – that was nearly half of my life.

I was pleased, when by week 3 the old me seemed to be back. I felt it proved that it was the treatment and I was determined to tell Dr Hickish that I wanted to stop the trial.

Part of the trial protocol meant having a CT scan every six weeks, so before my next chemo cycle I had a scan. When I went for pre-chemo, I was able to explain how I now definitely believed that the chemo was the cause of the extreme emotions I'd been experiencing, and that I wanted to change the drugs I was on. However, when Dr Hickish told me that my scan results were back and showed that after just two doses the cancer in my body had reduced by 69%, I was dumbstruck. That put a whole new spin on things. How could I even think about stopping a drug that was clearly working so well? But how could I consider putting myself and my family through the hell we'd been through already, every three weeks?

Thankfully Dr Hickish had an answer; he suggested reducing the dose by 20%. He felt that it would still be strong enough to effectively control the cancer, but the side effects should be much more manageable. I was so relieved that I didn't have to make an impossible decision, and thankfully the next cycle, although I felt emotional and teary, was nothing like what I'd experienced before – and no one got punched.

21

Another new routine

And so we started another routine – three weekly treatment, followed by a few days of extreme tiredness and extreme emotion, and then two weeks of feeling so much better and able to lead a fairly normal life.

I settled into life at the Day Centre, creating paintings and pottery, and enjoying the aromatherapy and reflexology massages that were available. I was amazed at how relaxing it was to sit and paint. I was able to totally lose myself in my work and not even think about cancer – which seems strange considering I was surrounded by people all with a terminal diagnosis.

It was at the Day Centre that I was told about a scheme being run by Toni & Guy hairdressers; they were offering a free consultation and then subsequent half price haircuts to people who had lost their hair through cancer treatment. My hair had started to grow back shortly after I'd finished my first course of chemotherapy, but I'd been too scared to grow it, because I was convinced I'd lose it again when I needed more treatment. Instead I continued to get the clippers out every couple of weeks and crop it really short. With the news that T-DM1 wouldn't cause hair loss, and after an upsetting incident when two lads had walked past Mel and I one evening and made the observation, "The skinhead must be a lesbian," I decided to make an appointment.

I had never been able to afford to splash out on high-end hairdressers before, and I felt a little intimidated by the trendy staff and 'posh' atmosphere, but I was soon relaxed by the massaging chairs and luxurious hair wash. Hannah, the manager, introduced herself as my new stylist and talked me through my options. She even managed to put a bit of shape into my very short hair. I went back every six weeks for my little bit of cut price luxury and soon had a lovely stylish hairstyle. Once I was happy with my new style I had to pay full-price, but by then I was hooked and I knew I would struggle to go back to my old hairdresser.

Having to have a CT scan every six weeks meant that I couldn't keep up the level of tension I'd experienced when being scanned less frequently, and once I'd had three or four positive scans that showed everything was stable, I began to relax a little. It was hard to get used to the idea that perhaps I had a future again and I felt some anger towards my doctors for being so negative in the first place. If I'd known I might have had a couple of years (or maybe even more) ahead of me, I think we would have done things very differently.

Mum had given up her job to be my carer, but I now wanted some independence back. It was hard to know what to do for the best, after all the girls had got used to her being around all the time and I still needed her when I'd had treatment. She didn't come over quite as often, but generally we decided not to change things too much because we didn't know how long it would be before things needed to change again – and we had become used to enjoying each other's company. I often think it is the day to day, cups of tea and shopping trips that are what the special memories are made of, rather than the grand gestures when everyone feels under pressure (that's not to say I don't enjoy the odd grand gesture of course).

The start of the new treatment coincided with me having been off work for eighteen months. My employers, Bournemouth Borough Council, had been very understanding and had told me that I didn't need to make any decisions about my position. However, I felt it was unfair to leave the team in limbo, waiting to see if I would come back. I also felt it would be better for me to make a proper break … I knew in my heart that I wouldn't be going back and there was no point in pretending I might. So I contacted HR to find out what my options were. It turned out that as long as Occupational Health approved it, I would be able to retire on health grounds.

I felt so pleased that I had listened to my parents when they told me I needed to opt into the pension scheme that the council offered, rather than continuing my somewhat cavalier attitude that the State would look after me when I got old. My doctors agreed that I would probably never be fit for work again, and so Occupational Health approved the retirement and I was able to claim my pension.

I had very mixed feelings about this – I felt it was a positive move in that I no longer felt I was letting people down by not being at work, and because I could relax into being a stay-at-home mum and concentrate on my treatment, but to be retired at 36 years old is a very strange feeling. I had been at a point in my career where things were changing – I was beginning to talk about the work I did to other adoption teams, and because of the research I had done, the Bournemouth model of 'Life Story' work was becoming best practice in other authorities. Now I would never know if I could have furthered my career and maybe qualified as a Social Worker – those possibilities were lost to me and I felt I'd lost part of who I was. However, I no longer needed to feel guilty when I went out shopping or for lunch whilst signed off sick, and I had an income again so I could afford those treats.

22

New friends

As time went on, my confidence grew and I began to feel more and more independent. When I'd been going through my low patch, Mel searched online to see what support was on offer. She came across an organisation called 'Breast Cancer Care', who promote themselves as being 'Here for anyone affected by breast cancer, bringing people together, providing support and campaigning for better standards of care'. Mel looked at their pages on secondary breast cancer and discovered that they ran courses and workshops for people living with secondary breast cancer, and specifically, one for younger women. I signed up and bought my train tickets, feeling excited and very nervous.

I remember Dad dropping me at the train station early one March morning. I checked I had my tickets about fifteen times and re-read my carefully copied out instructions on which platform I needed, at what time, and at which station.

The course was really interesting, informing us on the different medicines available, the pros and cons of drug trials, and effective ways to tackle fatigue, including a relaxation session with a guy who taught us how to self-hypnotise, which was rather amusing. There we were trying hard not to giggle – nine strangers, laid on the floor focusing on finding our 'happy place'.

A month later there was a follow up day, which concentrated on talking to family and friends about our illness, with a lot of focus on relating to children. It was very useful to hear other opinions and to have the things I'd already been doing reinforced as effective.

At the end of the second session, a few of us went for dinner on the South Bank and agreed to stay in touch. We formed a private group on Facebook and began to support each other in ways impossible for friends and family without cancer. Signing up for that workshop was one of the most positive things I've done, and having people in my life who are facing the same daily battles that I am, felt like finding the missing link.

I decided to stop seeing my counsellor. The work we'd done together had been very helpful in getting my head around a permanent, incurable illness that will probably take my life before I'm ready. She helped me come to terms with that and taught me to be kind to myself on the days that I couldn't come to terms with it – but it got to the point where we weren't going any further. I felt that each fortnight I would say the same stuff, cry about the same things and end up feeling emotionally drained after each session. There was no point in going over and over the same things and bringing me down each time. My counsellor had taught me ways to manage those feelings and so I felt she'd done her job. There have been times when it would have been good to talk to her again, but I have been able to draw on what she taught me in difficult times.

One of the most difficult and almost inevitable things that a cancer patient using support from other cancer patients has to deal with, is the loss of friends. After one or two old ladies at the Day Centre passed away, I realised that getting close to people I met there was a risky business. It was something I managed to avoid in the main, but then there was Pat. Pat managed to slip under my protective barrier and she became a good friend, a special lady, who I found myself caring for greatly.

The Day Centre caters for people with all sorts of cancers and other life threatening illnesses, but Pat and I were the only ones at the time with secondary breast cancer and, as we were both being treated at Bournemouth, we could compare notes about the doctors and nurses. Pat agreed with me that a new nurse was as useful as a 'chocolate teapot' and that her gum chewing and constant sniffing was hard to bear and very unprofessional. Pat let me moan about the arrogance of our registrar, but I knew deep down she had a soft spot for him, and it was when he took another job in a new hospital that she began to deteriorate. Whether this was a coincidence or whether his arrogance hid skills not shared by others, I don't know.

I sat next to Pat for lunch every week, and as the weeks went by she ate less and less – she really was wasting away in front of my eyes. Even in her last weeks she thought of others, making donations for my second hand book sale and lending me a book about Tenerife when I told her about my forthcoming holiday. She never complained about her illness or the pain she must have been in. Towards the end, when she was admitted to the hospice part of the Palliative Care Unit, she wouldn't see me because she didn't want to frighten me. When she died I was terribly sad, but was able to allow myself time to be sad and then feel thankful for her life and that I had been privileged enough to call her my friend.

Pat was an older lady, a grandmother, who had fought her battle for many years and had lived a full, happy life before cancer. The loss of friends from the Breast Cancer Care workshop was harder to deal with. When Ciaran died she was only 36 years old, two years younger than I was, and her little boy was only nine years old. She was an active campaigner, raising awareness of secondary breast cancer, making people realise that it's different to primary breast cancer and that patients have different needs. She lobbied Parliament, met with the Prime Minister and appeared on TV and radio, promoting her cause. She was in the middle of making a difference and her life was taken too soon. She was always so full of life – we had all met up a couple of months before she died and she didn't let on how ill she was, even then. She had wanted to go on the London Eye. "Us, together, on top of the world," were her words. The rest of us weren't keen and so it didn't happen. If we'd had an inkling then that we wouldn't see her again, we would have jumped at the opportunity, and I think it reminded us all to grab life by the balls a little more, rather than being sensible all the time.

Since then we have lost another of the group. Part of me feels I should be used to losing people I care about by now; sometimes I think I should delete their contact details and forget about them, and then I know that I couldn't do that, because although the pain was devastating and something I'll never get used to, I felt it because these people have played an important part in my life. They have picked me up when I was down, they have helped me feel less alone, and having them in my life was such a blessing. Losing two members of our group has brought the remaining group members closer. I feel they are a lifeline to feeling normal, and although I know that being close to them is a risky business, it's a risk I'm happy to take.

23

If you didn't laugh, you'd cry

Something that came up at the Breast Cancer Care workshop and is also reinforced weekly at the Day Centre, is that we need to care for ourselves as a whole. The Oncologists are finding drugs to fight the cancer, and in these times of effective drug treatment a terminal diagnosis usually means more than the six months to a year that used to be expected, in fact the word 'terminal' is being replaced with 'chronic' among medical professionals, demonstrating the way the illness can be managed for many years. Some of the ladies on the workshop and the people who attend the Day Centre have been living with cancer for seven, eight, even nine years. The future that I dared to wonder about in the last chapter, now seemed like a reality. I wasn't going to die any time soon and I needed to find a balance, getting back into a sensible routine and making the most of the times when I felt well.

I dropped a day at the Day Centre, just attending on a Monday and using the Wednesday to help out at Leah's school. It felt good to be doing something useful and worthwhile, and I know Leah loved having Mummy come into class every week to hear her and her friends reading.

I still had my hospital appointments and scans to keep me busy and didn't want to take on too much, but on the two weeks when the treatment wasn't affecting me, I began to lead a fairly full and active life again. I visited my friend Rhea in Oxford, I went on girlie weekends to Brighton, and Kev and I went to the Cotswolds and to Bath for romantic breaks. The weekend in Bath, using the Thermal Spa, was probably more romantic and relaxing than the trip to the Cotswolds, which included a day in Stratford-Upon-Avon. We decided that a row up the river would be a romantic adventure. It was not quite what we'd imagined, but at least we weren't the only ones shouting at each other about how to row and how to steer the boat.

Before I became a mother, I had lots of idealistic notions about how best to parent children. One strong view I'd held was that children shouldn't be taken abroad until they are about eight or nine years old. It's no fun for them on the plane when their ears hurt, nor should other passengers have to listen to a miserable toddler for the whole flight, then there's the heat to contend with when you get there and, basically, any parent who does it is just plain selfish.

I had formed this opinion whilst Kev and I were on our honeymoon, when a small child grizzled and kicked the back of my seat all the way to Corfu. Then when we were at the resort, there was another family, two parents and a three year old girl; they were always up and about before anyone else and at around midday, as it began to get hot, the mother would trudge back to their apartment with the little girl, whilst the father remained sprawled out by the pool. Sometimes the mother also bought him a pint of lager before leaving. Never would that happen to me.

Clearly, becoming a mother made me realise that there's no such thing as a perfect parent and everyone does things they previously thought they wouldn't, just to make life bearable. I had consoled myself with this thought when the only way I could get dressed in the mornings was to put Leah in front of the TV – despite my previous opinion that any parent who uses the TV as a babysitter doesn't deserve to be a parent at all.

I still thought that taking young children abroad probably wasn't the best idea, but when Kev and I talked about the things we should be doing now that we had our future back, one of those things was going abroad. Dr Hickish was all for it, so we arranged to go on the third week of my three weekly treatment cycle and delayed the next dose by a week so that I would be feeling as well as possible. I could only get travel insurance to cover anything other than cancer-related incidents, but we decided it was worth the risk.

We booked a week, self-catering in Puerto de Mogan, a quaint little fishing village on Gran Canaria. I researched the local health centres and English speaking doctors before we went with our just three-year-old and our nearly five-year-old. Guess what? The girls loved the flight. Going in November meant the heat was bearable, and when it was very hot we just stayed in the shade. We had the most amazing adventure … we were just a normal family on holiday together.

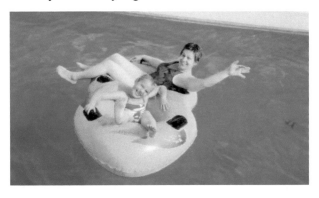

We made memories that will last forever; Kev, Leah and I kissed dolphins (Megan was too scared, so she watched) and Leah was chosen to appear in the show. She sat in a boat in front of more than eight hundred people, with dolphins jumping over her head. I cried. It was like the cancer wasn't there anymore. We went to a water park on one day and I went on most of the slides and made Kev and the girls hysterical with laughter by going in an Aquaball.

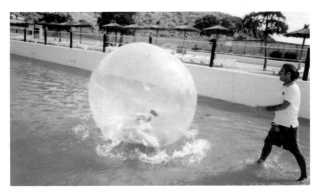

In the back of my mind I knew I was being reckless, due to my fragile bones, but I didn't want to worry about that on holiday, I wanted to take risks that I never would back in the UK. This was a holiday of a lifetime in a different way to Disney, because it was a normal family holiday, where lots of special things happened, rather than a holiday paid for by people who wanted us to enjoy our last months together, and with us knowing we had to make it special, because it might be our last holiday together.

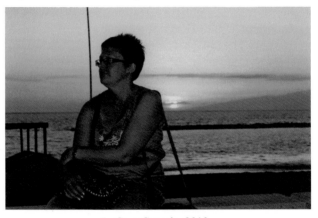

In Gran Canaria, 2010

I still look at the photos of Leah and the dolphins and cry. There was an incident that threatened to ruin the holiday, but we now look back on and laugh – the meeting with the timeshare salesman. We were approached by a surfer 'dude' who was handing out scratch cards, and surprisingly one of our cards won the gold prize. We were pointed in the direction of a hotel and told that if we just listened to a presentation we were guaranteed a prize. Kev, seeing the bottles of vodka and gin that were being carried out by other 'suckers', decided that it was worth listening, just for the free booze.

They were true to their word and gave us a drink, and the girls an ice-cream each, whilst a salesman from Merseyside hit us with his pitch. I switched off at the 'pay up front' bit, but Kev listened and let him talk. When he finished, he went to get us another drink, whilst we had a quick chat. I warned Kev that I wasn't afraid to 'play the cancer card' – perhaps not fair, but I guess there is an angry part of me that came out at the time.

When the salesman came back and asked what we thought, I confidently told him, "I'm afraid we're not in a position to make any kind of financial commitment at the moment." I knew he wouldn't accept just that, so when he asked why, I calmly said, "Because I have terminal cancer and don't know if we'll be able to take a holiday next year, let alone the year after."

I think he was actually speechless, which must be a fairly unusual position for a salesman on commission only. He gave me his condolences and whilst Kev and I finished our drinks, he chatted about the local area and life in Gran Canaria. I guess he felt he'd wasted over an hour on us and he decided on a last attempt. I was the next to be speechless when he came out with, "With all due respect Nikki, your family are going to take holidays when you're gone." I got up, told the girls to finish their ice-creams and, as I walked out, I said, "With all due respect to you, that's not something we're thinking about at the moment."

I know that my remark must have made him defensive, but I was amazed he could be so insensitive, especially in front of the girls. Kev followed on my heels, but not without getting his bottle of gin on the way out.

It can be incredible the things people say, I'm sure not maliciously, but just without thinking. Not long after I'd retired from work and just before we went to Gran Canaria, we went out on a Saturday evening and I bumped into a friend I'd not seen for about a year. We had lots to catch up on; we laughed about how lucky I am to be retired from work, we joked about my leisurely lifestyle and how 'it's alright for some' that I'm off on holiday again next week. Not once did we mention the tedious and often traumatic hospital visits, we didn't talk about the way I have to treasure every happy moment with the girls or how I sometimes lie in bed at night worrying how they will cope growing up without me. The conversation ended with him telling me how cushy my life is.

Then there was the guest of honour at a Cancer Research UK ball I attended, who was privately fighting his own cancer battle. He told me how brave I was exposing my near bald head,

"… but haven't you ever thought of going down the wig route."
Actually, no I hadn't, not that it was any of his business.

There are the people who tell me I can cure myself if I just eat such and such, because they know someone whose brother's wife's uncle had 'exactly the same as you and they're better now just because of this diet.' I know they mean well, but I need to live my life my way and make my own decisions.

There's an email game that does the rounds every now and again, called Cancer Catch-phrase Bingo, and it lists all the things people commonly say to cancer patients and you have to see how high you score – you have to laugh about these things or else you'd cry.

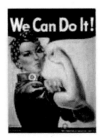

Cancer catchphrase bingo

Bored by platitudes, tilted heads and fake empathy?
You need CanDoCancer Bingo!
Oh yes my friends, finally put out this handy pocked-sized grid and tick off the cancer catchphrases when they are addressed to you.
Anything similar also counts.
Let us know when you've completed your card and we'll promise to let you buy the wine at our next event.
You're all so inspirational dahlings!

You're so inspirational!	I'm in awe of you!	Anything involving the word 'icon'.	My friend's neighbour's cousin died of that.
Any war metaphors (fight, battle)	Be positive	You'll be fine. I know because my friend had it.	But you look fine?
Kylie Minogue references.	What do you think you did to get that?	Black grapes cure that (Other foodstuffs also permitted)	Are you cured now?
I had a lump once, but it turned out to be ok.	Is there anything I can do?	Sudden change of subject	You're **sooo** brave.
Yes, you could die of it, but then any of us could get hit by a bus tomorrow.	Oh, so do you get to have perky new boobs? (Also, eye flickering in that area)	So how ARE you? (Must be accompanied by tilted head)	Maybe it's a good opportunity to loo at how you're living your life?

24

Relationships

Friends come and go in life, and when you have cancer they more often go. Actually that's not entirely true, I have been supported by the most amazing friends and have gained some new friends who have enriched my life enormously, but I have had friends who have just upped and left because they couldn't cope with my illness – and it bloody hurts.

I am fortunate enough to belong to a large, close-knit family; my mum and my sister Mel are actively involved in my daily life and offer me tremendous emotional support, my dad and brother are the strong, silent types, but I know they are always there for me and would do anything I asked of them. Uncle Steve drives me wherever I want to go, from hospital appointments to massage sessions, to trips to London. He'll collect prescriptions for me, and on his days off work he rings to see if there's anything I want him to do for me. If Uncle Steve isn't around, his wife, Jan, or Auntie Cilla (the wife of my uncle who died) will be, so I never need worry if I don't feel up to driving.

Since I was pregnant with Leah, I have been a member of an on-line parenting message board, and although we started off as mums talking about our kids, we soon became friends who shared everything from painful periods to embarrassing crushes. We have supported members through miscarriage, bereavement and relationship breakdown, and they have supported me through my cancer journey. There is always someone on-line, even in the middle of the night (crying babies keep people awake). They have been able to support me in ways that my family and 'real life' friends couldn't, because they are a step removed. When I was first diagnosed, most of us had never met. I was overwhelmed when, after mentioning I should have 'Meet the

Chicks' on my bucket list, a party in Bournemouth was organised.

Rhea, the other girls from university and I meet as often as we can. Sometimes it can be a year between our get togethers, but we always have a wonderful time and it feels as if no time at all has been lost. Rhea and I are especially close, Rhea being one of Leah's Supporting Adults. We sometimes meet up without the others to spend time together and with our children.

Rhea is probably the person who knows me best in the world – having lived together for two years and shared many a bottle of wine in the kitchen of our tiny basement flat, we told each other everything. Our busy lives keep us apart more than we'd like, but she is still a very special friend.

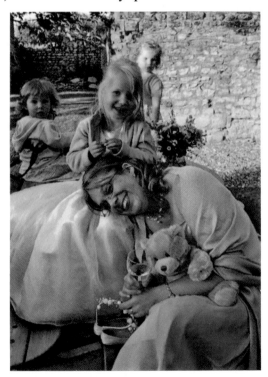

Megan, Leah and Nikki at Rhea's wedding, June 2008

Keren is my 'Mummy Friend'. We met when Leah and her daughter, Joni, were babies, and we have since gone on to have second daughters born on the same day. (She now has gone on to have a third daughter.) We meet up with the children as often as we can. Keren has been a great support in the way she has the girls for sleepovers for me, keeping things normal for them and always knows the right thing to say, often just a text saying, 'Chin up.'

I'm sure there are people I've forgotten, but I need to end this little tribute by talking about Cathy, the person I've been friends with since primary school, the person who is always at the end of a telephone, the person who looks after the girls for a weekend "because I love having them". Cathy is my best friend and has been the best of friends to me throughout my whole life – cancer is just another of life's hiccups.

So those are the friends who have stood by me. Unfortunately, there have been others who 'couldn't handle it'. I'm not going to go into detail, but it has been very painful the way some people have just removed themselves from our lives completely, people who really should have known better. At first I was very angry, but now I just feel sad – and sad for them too, because they've missed out on so much, missed out on our girls growing into beautiful little people, missed out on special events that my cancer has allowed us to experience. When I'm being particularly generous, I kind of understand and think if they really can't handle it, then it's best they keep away, but most of the time I feel bereft of our friendships. I feel so lucky that I have enough friends to see me through and I hope that should those that didn't stick by me ever find themselves in my situation, they will have good friends who stick by them.

The other relationship that has been hugely affected is my marriage. Statistics show that husbands of terminally ill wives are more likely to leave, than the wives of terminally ill men. Kev has stuck by me, despite the fact that at times it's been very hard for him. During darker times he has commented that he's trapped, because everyone would call him rude names if he left me. There have been times when he's distanced himself from me and we've gone for weeks, only speaking when it's absolutely necessary. We've had some real humdinger rows, when things have been said that never should have been, but we have also experienced some wonderfully close times when we have shared everything. Our whole future was ripped away from us in one day. We had always talked about retiring to somewhere hot, and that dream was gone overnight. Kev suddenly had an awful lot of pressure put on him: the pressure of a sick wife, of people judging his treatment of me, having to be around more, feeling he could never be ill because he'd never be as ill as me, and obviously, deep fear that he was going to lose me and become a single parent.

I don't think we've really dealt with it – we've muddled along. We did go for three sessions with Relate, after a particularly bad time when I really thought things were over between us. Sitting in a room with a stranger between us, allowed us to say the things we were feeling without it turning into a huge row. Kev was able to tell me that he felt he couldn't make plans for the future in case I got upset that they didn't include me, I was able to reassure him that hearing him say that was such a relief to me, because it proved he was coming to terms with a future without me and had some sort of plan in place. He told me that he felt in a 'no win' situation, because if we split up he'd never be forgiven for leaving a sick wife, but when he has talked to his friends about how bad things have got between us he has worried that they think he's only with me out of pity and because he stands to inherit a fair bit of insurance money when I die. I was able to reassure him that he'd get that money anyway, because it's to go towards looking after Leah and Megan, which he would do whether we were together or not.

We cried a lot during these sessions, which was therapeutic, but the main thing we took away from the sessions was the importance of communication. If only Kev had told me his worries earlier, he wouldn't have felt the need to distance himself so much, and if I were more open to such discussions, then again he wouldn't have felt so lonely and unable to talk to me. We agreed to listen more.

25

The trial drug

The trial drug kept my cancer stable for two years and eight months, and during that time I became used to managing the side effects and trying to make the most of my life. Apart from the three to four days immediately after treatment, I was well and mainly enjoyed my life. We enjoyed another family holiday abroad, this time to Tenerife.

Kev's nan sadly passed away, and with the money they inherited, his parents invested in two caravans in Weymouth, on the site where we had stayed previously. They used one to spend their summers in and rented the other out, keeping two weeks free for us and two weeks free for Leanne and her family. It meant some lovely holidays, where the girls were able to spend quality time with their other grandparents.

After a nasty infection at the site of my tunnel line, I spent two days and nights in hospital and had to have the line removed. Thankfully, because of the length of time the line had been in, my veins had recovered enough to be used again successfully for several months. By the time they began to play up again, my hospital had trained their nurses in the use of portacaths. A portacath is a small port inserted just below the skin, with a catheter connecting it to a vein. It works in a similar way to the tunnel line, but being under the skin the risk of infection is minimal, which is beneficial in itself, but also means the patient is allowed to go swimming. I was thrilled this was now an option for me and asked to be referred.

Remembering my experience with the tunnel line insertion, I asked to be properly sedated. The doctor (a different one to usual) assured me it wouldn't be necessary, that a small relaxant was all that I'd need. I assured him that wasn't the case, but he wouldn't listen, saying if I experienced pain during the procedure he'd be able to top up what he'd given me. I was very unhappy and therefore very tense. As soon as he started operating, I complained that I didn't like it and I wanted to be asleep. I know I was becoming very distressed, but it wasn't until I screamed in pain that he gave me something stronger. The result being I experienced the whole procedure and then fell asleep in recovery. I was so upset. I felt angry that they hadn't listened to me and angry with myself for not making my position clearer before the procedure started. I even felt angry that it had been a different doctor and not the usual one, who understands my needs a bit better. Imagine my shock and upset when I read in my local paper about a popular hospital doctor dying in tragic circumstances on September 25th and saw the name of the doctor who had inserted all my tunnel lines. September 25th was the day I had my portacath fitted. Doctors aren't meant to die; they are meant to be indestructible aren't they? I felt very shaken by the news and made the decision then that if I need another 'simple procedure' I will insist on a general anaesthetic from the start.

Traditionally, chemotherapy treatments are a course of six treatments that make you very sick and then you get better – or die. When my treatment went on for so much longer, people who had been very supportive in the beginning began to think we were exaggerating things. The situation at Kev's work became very difficult; he had been taken out of his previous role and was assisting his manager, on the same salary as others with far more responsibility. He was allowed to come in late and drop things at a moment's notice if I needed him. Some of his colleagues felt this was unfair and began to treat him very badly, spreading rumours that he was lying about my treatment and on one occasion actually telling him during a staff meeting that he was 'an absolute joke'. He knew that the friend he had worked with when he was self-employed, had lots of work on, so he handed in his notice and went to join him. The first job he had was refurbishing a rest home. The owner of the rest home was impressed with Kev and took him on permanently as a maintenance man. It meant less hours and also less money, but Kev was so much more relaxed, and happier – and we saw more of him. I was very upset about the experience in his previous job, although I could understand why people felt he was being treated favourably and it wasn't fair – that wasn't Kev's fault and it certainly wasn't a position we'd choose to be in.

For a while I felt paranoid that others may be feeling that way about us, that perhaps I didn't deserve my benefits and should be going out to work. Mum and Kev gave me a talking to and I soon realised that if people did feel like that it was their problem, not mine. I knew what I was capable of and what I was going through, and that was enough to be dealing with, without worrying what other people thought.

As things seemed to be going well and were continuing to do so, I decided I needed to be more active. I had become very unfit since my diagnosis and, although the medical advice is that gentle exercise is so good for you – especially as a cancer patient, I chose to ignore that advice and wallow in laziness. As I came round to thinking that I wasn't going to die anytime soon, I felt I needed to be as fit and healthy as possible, to have a better chance of living longer, so it was with interest that I saw a sign on my local church notice board advertising a 'gentle aerobic exercise class'. I thought it would be perfect as a warm up, to see what I was capable of.

Mum agreed to come with me and we went along the following Friday morning. We paid our admission to a rather large lady of about seventy years of age, who was sat in the doorway. As we went in and took our coats off, we cast our eyes around the room. If I hadn't been there, Mum would have been the youngest by about twenty years. If we hadn't been spotted at that moment by Leah's Brownie leader, we probably would have made our escape, but alas, we felt we had to stick it out.

When the rather large, seventy year old took her position at the front of the room and began to introduce the class, I could feel the giggles building up inside me. She explained that after the warm-up there would be a dance section, before a toning session using chairs, then another dance session, before the cool down. I felt ashamed of my mocking and my fitness level, when the warm-up made my legs shake. Before my illness I had been fairly fit, and before children I had been very fit, using the gym, running, swimming and exercise DVDs. I was shocked at how little I could now do.

Then came the dance section. Mum and I watched in amazement as fifteen elderly ladies shook their stuff to Lady Gaga. However, things started to go wrong when the routine became more complicated, people started to bump into each other and at one point the instructor had to stop to remember the moves, skip back the CD and try again. It was hilarious; I think I did the whole routine with a bemused smirk on my face.

What finally finished me off was over-hearing a conversation between Mum and an old lady, and seeing Mum's face afterwards.

Old lady – "Hello dear, what's your name?"
Mum – "My name's Ann. What's yours?"
Old lady – "Oh, I'm fine, thank you dear."

Thankfully, the cool down was just coming to an end, so we were able to make our escape and crash riotously down the stairs. We stuck to beach walks after that …

26

What makes me a woman?

As a woman there are many things that define me, and living with breast cancer changes that definition. I was very fortunate not to need a mastectomy, and so still have the breasts that in the past I had always been very fond of. The feeling of ambivalence I now feel towards them is a little upsetting but, in the big scheme of things, not really something to complain about.

In the summer of 2012 I had a pregnancy scare. My periods had returned about six months after I finished the first course of chemo, and they had been regular since then. Dr Hickish had told me my chances of falling pregnant were very slim, but due to the trial it was very important that I didn't. We were on holiday in Weymouth, in the new caravan that Kev's parents had bought. The day my period was due, it crossed my mind that it was unusual for me to be late; perhaps I'd marked the wrong day in my diary. The next day I was a bit more concerned, I looked back over my diary and noted that I had been as regular as clockwork for the past six months. By the third day I was really trying hard not to panic. I mentioned it to Kev and he told me to try to forget about it until we got home. That night I lay in bed worrying.

I have always been pretty opinionated and have a strong sense of right and wrong, but abortion is something I've never got my head around. I do believe it is the woman's right to choose – but it doesn't sit easy with me, and I always thought that no matter what my circumstances it is something I, personally, would never be able to do … and now it was looking like a definite possibility. If I had been stupid enough to let myself get pregnant, there was no way on earth I could have the baby. Firstly, I would have to stop my treatment, which would be detrimental to my health and therefore the baby's. Secondly, it was hard enough to think of leaving Leah and Megan; there was no way I could leave Kev as a single father of three. And finally, I'd had a CT scan the week before, when they always ask if you could be pregnant, because the radiation can damage an unborn baby, so the chances were I'd already done untold damage anyway. I couldn't even think about it as a potential baby.

The week dragged by. I kept going to the toilet with my fingers crossed and, although I put on a cheerful face for the girls, it was the longest holiday of my life. I didn't want to buy a pregnancy test, because with both my previous pregnancies I'd tested when my period had been four or five days late and it had been negative. I hadn't got a positive result until I was seven or eight days late. The Monday after the holiday I had a pre-chemo appointment with Dr Hickish. Mum usually came with me to these appointments, but because it was school holidays she was looking after the girls for me. I was glad I'd have the opportunity to pop to Tesco without her knowing, to buy a test. I'd decided it was time, and I needed to know.

I felt very tense at my appointment. We ran through the usual questions; How was I feeling? Not bad. Any nausea? No more than usual. Any pain? No. Then he asked if there was anything else bothering me. I burst into tears and it all came pouring out. Dr Hickish was very kind, but stressed how important it was that we find out immediately. He called a nurse in and asked her to get a pregnancy test for me. It was humiliating; I felt like a silly school girl. And then it was all over … the test was negative. I cried again, this time with relief. I pulled myself together and asked Dr Hickish to refer me to a gynaecologist to be sterilized.

The referral for sterilization had to come from my GP and I had to have a counselling appointment first. Dr Mitchell had to ensure that I fully understood the implications of female sterilization. He explained that male sterilization was thirty times more likely to be successful and twenty times less likely to have post-op complications, due to it being a less invasive procedure. I knew from past conversations that Kev really wasn't keen to consider having the snip himself, and the idea of an operation really didn't bother me, but it was more than that, Kev was only 35 years old at the time, after I'm gone it's quite likely he'll meet someone new and perhaps want to have a family with them. For me, my baby making days were well and truly over. As far as I was concerned there was no discussion to be had, it was me having the operation.

I have never been broody before. Kev wanted us to have a baby and convinced me it was a good idea, then when we'd had Leah I knew I didn't want her to be an only child, so we had Megan. I had never felt that deep desire to be pregnant and have a tiny baby – until I was booked in to be sterilized. It was really strange, there were pregnant women everywhere I looked, or seemed to be anyway. I could imagine being pregnant, I could almost feel the baby inside me and that feeling in your womb when a baby breastfeeds – I could feel that too. It was that deep desire, no, more than that, deep desperation to have a baby inside me or in my arms. It was a horrible experience and I'm certain if I'd been having the operation for any reason other than the fact that I simply couldn't have another baby under any circumstances, I would have changed my mind.

The operation went reasonably smoothly; although at the time I had a portacath fitted (the port situated under the skin for receiving intravenous medication) and the anaesthetist wasn't happy using it, so he tried to cannulate me for the general anaesthetic. Needless-to-say he couldn't find a vein. He decided to put me to sleep using gas through a mask and then insert the cannula when I was already asleep, so that he could put it at the base of my thumb (a vein I had refused to let him use, because I had passed out in pain the last time someone tried to use that site).

The next thing I knew, I was in the recovery room feeling very tender and hungry. A nurse brought me pain relief, marmite on toast and a cup of tea. Mum and Uncle Steve came to get me, and when I got home I took myself off to bed, where I slept until the next morning. Now, I know I'd had fairly major surgery, but for some reason I hadn't factored in recovery time, and I certainly hadn't considered how it would affect me emotionally. I thought it would cure my broodiness, but instead I felt that I'd lost my femininity, I'd lost what defines me as a woman – the ability to have children. I realise how self-centred and indulgent that must sound, especially as I've been fortunate enough to have had two healthy babies, but I felt bereaved.

I tried to keep myself busy to take my mind off things and so made the recovery process longer. I experienced severe stomach cramps and heavy bleeding for well over a week. Once I realised I needed to take it easy, I was feeling better within a couple of days.

Thankfully, the emotions I experienced initially, passed after a week or so, and I soon realised I had made the right decision; I no longer had to go through the embarrassment of explaining how I knew I wasn't pregnant whenever I had a scan, and I didn't have to panic every time my period was late, which became a more common occurrence as time went on.

27

Back on the rollercoaster

Although I had definitely become more relaxed, and possibly a little complacent, about my six weekly CT scans, of course it was always in the back of my mind that one day the news would be bad. The six week summer holiday of 2012 was wonderful, despite the weather not being fabulous, and the girls and I, either with Mum or with friends, had lots of day trips.

We enjoyed Brownsea Island with Keren and her girls, the Bournemouth Air Festival with Cathy and her children, as well as time in Weymouth with my brother, Matt, and nephews, Jay and Leo. Mum and I looked after Thom on several occasions, as by now Mel was expecting again – this time twins.

However, despite this very special time, I had noticed that it was taking me longer to recover from my treatment – only by a day or so, but still a noticeable difference. Also my emotions seemed to go a bit crazy, nothing like it had been at the beginning of this treatment, but lots of uncontrollable crying, and on some days feeling that I really needed a good cry, wanting the release it offers and just not being able to let go.

The six weekly scan routine was so relaxed that I didn't even have an outpatient appointment with Dr Hickish to discuss the results, I would either be told at my next pre-chemo appointment or a research nurse would ring to let me know all was fine. On October 3rd 2012, I had a pre-chemo appointment with one of Dr Hickish's registrars, and she told me that my scan had shown some enlarged lymph nodes in the back of my stomach cavity. She told me not to worry, because they were only very slightly enlarged and it could easily have been caused by an infection or virus. I came away feeling a little shaken. I had read a report online about the success of the T-DM1 trial and how for many HER2 positive breast cancer patients it has been effective, having also extended their lives. At that point in time I had been on T-DM1 for thirty one months.

Note on the EMILIA trial: '... the objective response rate (i.e. per cent of patients in whom the tumour shrinks appreciably - there being a strict definition of this) was 43.6 percent versus 30.8 for the standard therapy with a 5 month improvement in median overall survival.

I saw Dr Hickish at my next pre-chemo appointment, three weeks later, and mentioned the scan results to him. He looked surprised that I had been told, and I believe if I had seen him at my last appointment he wouldn't even have mentioned the enlarged lymph nodes at this stage. I felt reassured by this, but couldn't shake the article I had read from my mind – surely my time on this trial was up and I was fortunate that it had been so successful for me.

After my next scan, I waited anxiously for the appointment at which I would get the results. I saw the registrar again and she told me that the lymph nodes were further enlarged and this time she felt it was a more significant progression. She told me that she'd have to discuss the results with Dr Hickish and he'd decide the next course of action. As an afterthought, she added that he 'may still think it's insignificant', but neither of us believed that. She told me that she would ring me the next day to let me know what he said.

Despite the fact I had been expecting this news, it still came as a shock. My legs turned to jelly and when I got home I fainted. When I'd calmed down, I thought some more about it and felt that maybe this wasn't a disaster after all. I had been becoming fed-up on the T-DM1, with the side effects becoming more difficult to manage, so perhaps a change in treatment would be good for me.

The next day came and went and I heard nothing. I was feeling very anxious and the waiting was very stressful. The next day, when I still hadn't heard anything, I rang Ward 10 to see if I could find anything out. The registrar wasn't available, but the admin clerk told me that there was a MDT (Multi-Disciplinary Team) meeting the next day and my case was down to be discussed; he was sure I'd hear something tomorrow.

Hearing about the MDT meeting brought mixed feelings, it was good that they were considering my case properly and looking at all options … but it must be serious if it needed to be discussed by lots of experts.

I didn't hear anything the next day either. I was feeling very angry by now; did they not know how scared and anxious I was feeling? I kept playing different scenarios over and over in my mind; maybe they'd decided the lymph nodes weren't significant, so weren't worried, not realising how worried I was, or maybe the news was so bad they needed to see me face-to-face and so were waiting until they could offer me an appointment. All sorts of possibilities went through my mind over what turned out to be five days, before I heard anything.

On the Friday (the initial appointment being the previous Monday) I phoned Ward 10 in tears, and thankfully I spoke to a nurse who really seemed to get it. She promised me she'd get someone to call me back today – even if it were just her to tell me she couldn't find anyone.

Five hours later, I heard from a different registrar. She told me that the enlarged lymph nodes could be something to do with soft tissue and that I shouldn't be worrying, that it was up to Dr Hickish to worry and make the decisions. She said Dr Hickish would be in touch when it was time for me to know something. This doctor had a strong accent and I struggled to follow her, but I understood that she was telling me I shouldn't be worrying. I felt such a mixture of emotions, exhausted from all the crying and worrying, confused about what the enlarged lymph nodes meant and very angry with the doctors for worrying me in the first place and then not ringing back to put my mind at rest. It all made me feel that I was being a drama queen, making such a fuss over what could still turn out to be nothing. Mum was worried that I was going to sink into that deep depression again and kept bullying me to get up and do things, but I just didn't have the motivation or inclination.

Then I watched Children In Need. Thankfully, Leah and Megan had gone to bed when they showed a video clip of a family coming to terms with a mother's terminal breast cancer diagnosis and subsequent death – I sobbed and sobbed. But it did help me put things into perspective. This journey can be so difficult at times, but I still have so much to fight for and so much to enjoy before I can even consider rolling over and giving up.

On Monday 19th November, I received the news that the cancer was spreading in the back of my abdomen … only in a small way, but enough to warrant a change in treatment. I was given an appointment for the following Monday to discuss my treatment options. I felt relieved that I finally had some answers, angry that I had been messed around for a whole week and gutted that my wonderful trial drug had stopped working.

Kev decided that now was a great time to start major building work on our flat. We had acknowledged that we were growing out of the space that we had, but we weren't able to move. Even though our mortgage had been paid off, the equity wasn't enough to buy somewhere bigger, we would have to borrow more, which we didn't feel comfortable doing, given our situation. The flat wasn't particularly well designed and had a tiny kitchen, only really big enough for one person. I felt sad that it was impossible to accommodate the girls and so their only experience of cake making and cooking experiments had happened at Mum's.

Over the time we'd lived here, every few months we would talk about ways of making the kitchen bigger, but had never quite come up with the best way to do it. Kev would have happily built an extension, but I didn't want the upheaval or expense. During our latest chat, I half-jokingly said, "Why don't we put the bathroom in the hall and knock the wall down between the kitchen and current bathroom?" Kev's face lit up and out came his tape measure and notepad. He started taking measurements and making sketches. "It would fit," he told me.

He explained that we may need to lose the bath and just have a shower room, and that we'd lose a hallway width of our bedroom, but the benefits of having a kitchen twice the size would outweigh that loss. I agreed, but immediately started panicking about the mess and chaos this work would involve. I made Kev promise that we would wait until after Christmas.

The day I got the news that the cancer had grown and I needed to change my treatment (Nov 19th) Kev knocked a great big hole in our bedroom wall. Perhaps this was his way of coping with my news? The work got underway, the girls and I spent a few weekends either at Cathy's house or at Mum and Dad's and, although it was chaotic and very stressful, it was worth it when it was finished and our living space was so much more efficient.

My appointment came round after a long week of worrying. I kept coming back to the idea that if my cancer had beaten this 'super drug', the best treatment available, then what chance did any other treatment have?

The actual appointment felt a bit of an anti-climax. Dr Hickish said he felt the best option for me would be Capecitabine and Lapatinib, the two drugs that were the other arm of the trial. I had done a bit of research on them when I was waiting to hear which arm of the trial I had been selected for and I also knew that a couple of my friends from the Breast Cancer Care course had experience of them. The side effects included anaemia, nausea, vomiting, diarrhoea, soreness and redness of hands and feet, tiredness, headaches, indigestion, stomach cramps, mouth ulcers and constipation. It sounded horrendous, but I also knew that Caroline (from the Breast Cancer Care course) had continued working through her time on Capecitabine, and Dr Hickish reassured me that although there were side effects, very few people experienced all of them and usually only experience them mildly, so I didn't worry too much. I was told that before I could begin the new regime I had to allow the T-DM1 to leave my body, so I was given another appointment for three weeks' time to go back and finalise things. In the meantime I would have to have an MRI to check my bones were as good as they appeared on the CT.

I went home and updated my Facebook status, so that all my friends and family, who I knew would have been thinking of me, knew how the appointment had gone. Of course, everyone thought it was great news – mild side effects, keeping my hair etc. I knew it was all true, but I just didn't feel that way – I still had cancer, I still had to have treatment and all I could think was that it was hugely unfair.

28

Another treatment regime

Approximately three weeks later, on a Thursday, I had a pre-chemo appointment in preparation for starting Capecitabine and Lapatinib. The doctor noticed that I had a cough, so prescribed antibiotics, saying that I wouldn't be able to start the new drugs on Monday if I was still coughing. That weekend I had a really upset stomach, Mel said it was probably the antibiotics, but I felt sure it was anxiety. I had so many feelings and concerns buzzing around my head. It was strange; I was just as worried about being well as I was about suffering side effects. Knowing Caroline's experience, I was scared about how I was going to fill my days if I suffered no side effects; I was scared I'd lose my benefits if I was well in myself and I had become so used to being looked after by Mum and everyone else that I wasn't sure if I'd cope again, being independent.

I had been living with this illness for just over five years, which in itself seemed quite impossible; I wasn't supposed to be alive any more, let alone getting better. But then on the other hand, what if I did suffer the side effects? The sore hands and feet sounded horrible; the doctor I saw at pre-chemo had said if they became cracked and raw I'd need to soak them in salt water to prevent infection. I was going around in circles, not knowing what to think.

The new chemo regime involved fifteen huge tablets a day; five Lapatinib before I got up in the morning, then wait an hour to have breakfast and take five Capecitabine, and then five more Capecitabine with my evening meal. This was for the first twenty one days, and then I would have a week off the Capecitabine, before starting it all again. I was still feeling a bit shell-shocked and was thankful the girls had already broken up from school for the Christmas holidays, so I didn't have to think about getting up and doing the school run in those early days of the new treatment.

It was at this time that Community Cancer Nurse (CCN) Nikki came into my life. It was felt that, because my new treatment was in tablet form, I didn't need to go to the hospital for it. I was still taking the Zoledronate intravenously, but this could be administered at home. I would have to go for a pre-chemo appointment once a month, for a blood test, weight check, blood pressure check and chat with a doctor – other than that it was all done at home. It felt fantastic; for the past five years I had spent so much time at the hospital and now (apart from three monthly scans) I only had to go once a month. Nikki would pick my prescription up from the hospital pharmacy, she could prescribe any drugs that I'd forgotten to ask for and she was at the end of the telephone if I had any problems or queries. I soon began to wonder how I'd managed without her for so long and felt very lucky to have such a fantastic service available to me.

It took about a week for the side effects to kick in – Christmas morning and the diarrhoea started. Thankfully, I felt fine in myself so was able to enjoy Christmas, but by New Year's Eve I was in my GP surgery with what felt like flu, and the cough that I'd had was back with a vengeance. Dr Mitchell explained that they don't usually prescribe antibiotics for flu, but as they seemed to help when I had the cough, he would prescribe another course. That New Year's Eve, for the first time in my adult life I was in bed asleep before the bells chimed midnight – even a three week old Leah hadn't stopped me seeing the New Year in, but this bug really knocked me for six.

Kev was feeling a bit under the weather too so he didn't mind an early night. The girls, however, were very disappointed. They asked if they could stay up without us. We compromised and pretended it was midnight at ten o'clock; we got the champagne flutes out, filled with orange juice, and we toasted the New Year then packed ourselves off to bed.

Over the next few months I really struggled. I had to change the timing of taking the tablets, because taking five tablets first thing in the morning made me sick. I started to get up, eat breakfast, then take the Capecitabine, and then I would wait until half past eleven to take the Lapatinib and not have lunch until after twelve thirty. I found it suited me better that way, although I still experienced vomiting. It was very frustrating, because there was no pattern or cycle as to when it would happen. I also found that eating my main meal at lunchtime worked better for me – especially if Mum cooked it.

However, one morning Mum phoned to see how I was, we chatted for a while and then she mentioned that she'd saved me some of their roast beef dinner from the previous day and that she'd bring it over when she came. I had to drop the phone and rush to the bathroom, where I was violently sick. Mum still brought the meal over and by lunchtime I was not only able to eat it, but enjoy it.

Taking a Metaclopramide (anti-sickness drug) half an hour before eating also helped keep the sickness under control, although I did have a constant feeling of nausea. As well as sickness, I also experienced a lot of diarrhoea. Again, there was no pattern to when this would occur, and the worse thing was that it would sometimes happen at night and I wouldn't always wake up. It was awful, I felt devastated that this was happening to me, I couldn't stop thinking, 'I'm thirty eight for goodness sake, not some incontinent old biddy'. I felt that the doctors weren't really interested. "It's just one of those things" they'd say, but to me it was a massive thing. If I felt I had a gripey tummy before I went to bed, I would wear an incontinence pad, but I didn't always feel unwell before it happened, so did have accidents.

The worst occasion was one night when Kev was away. Megan came in to my bedroom in the middle of the night with leg pain (she often experienced 'growing pains' at that time). As I woke up I realised that I was in a mess, so had to dash to the bathroom. She was crying in pain and followed me, not understanding why I wasn't dealing with her. She was so upset when she saw the state I was in – no child should see their mother like that. She was getting more and more distressed as I tried to clean myself up. It was the worst experience and really made me wonder if it was all worthwhile.

The trouble was that during the first two months on this treatment I had the flu as well and I ended up taking three courses of antibiotics, so it was impossible to tell if it was them causing the upset stomach or the chemo. As a result I was reluctant to change the dose of the chemo at that stage. After a particularly bad bout of diarrhoea, lasting several days, the doctor decided to extend the break from the Capecitabine from the usual week to a fortnight. I was amazed at how well I felt by the end of the second week off. It reassured me that it was the Capecitabine making me feel so awful.

Two weeks earlier, I had been sleeping a lot (up to eighteen hours a day some days) and lacking in motivation to do anything, and that was as well as the sickness and diarrhoea. Nikki (CCN) thought that I would benefit from a lower dose of the Capecitabine, but Dr Hickish felt that as long as I had a longer break when the side effects were too much, I should stay on the dose I was taking. I ended up having several breaks; on occasion my feet became so sore, cracked and bleeding that it was painful to walk, and when the diarrhoea was particularly bad I would have a longer break. I noticed each time how much better I felt during that second week off and wondered if it was worth all the suffering.

Then I had a CT scan ... the drugs were working. That night I wrote in my diary, 'This hell has been worth it.'

But was it ... really? I would wake up around ten o'clock in the morning, drag myself onto the sofa, where I would doze until lunchtime. After lunch, I would take myself back to the sofa and watch mind-numbing daytime television, have another sleep whilst Mum went to pick the girls up from school, then I would try to spend a couple of hours with the girls; chatting, reading or watching television (nothing too strenuous), before heading to bed at around eight o'clock. That's a description of a worst possible day – but they happened and fairly frequently.

I was able to force myself to do things if it was something I really wanted to do. Our week at the caravan in Weymouth thankfully fell during an extended break, so I was well enough to enjoy it – as long as I didn't get up too early and could have a nap mid-afternoon if I needed to. It really was no fun at all, for any of us.

29

An impossible decision

For just over four months I felt like I was just existing. It seemed that I was never leaving the flat; in reality I did continue to attend my writing group every fortnight, every six weeks I had my massage with Stacey, and I occasionally went out for lunch with an old work colleague. These were things I had always enjoyed doing, and with encouragement from Mum and Kev I forced myself to keep them up, but most of the time I stayed in and sat on the sofa, rarely even getting dressed.

Then two things happened. First of all I turned thirty nine, and Cathy gave me a beautiful handmade scrapbook that I decided I would use to record my fortieth year, a year of opportunities and new experiences, and so I came up with a list of things I wanted to do before I was forty:-

- See a show
- Go to a concert
- Ride a horse
- Try a new spa treatment
- Finish my book and get on the route to publishing
- Visit a new city
- Paint a picture
- Wear a pair of killer heels
- Try a new craft
- Volunteer
- Karaoke

I did wonder how I was going to achieve all of this, but felt inspired to have some goals, and I think I also knew deep down that the agony had to come to an end one way or another.

The second thing that happened was a long, tearful chat with

Lynn, a Community Cancer Nurse who was filling in for Nikki. I cried and talked for over two hours, telling her how low I was feeling, how I felt so tired all the time and didn't have the energy or inclination to do anything, how I felt sad for the girls and a nuisance to Mum and Kev. I told her I felt I had no quality of life. She listened to me and suggested I take a longer break from the Capecitabine, instead of starting the next cycle the next day I should leave it another week to give my body more of a chance to recover.

She also said I should return to the Macmillan Day Centre. I had stopped going during my time on the trial, when my life had levelled out, I wasn't suffering side effects and my emotions had settled. At that time I had found going to the Day Centre was actually doing me more harm than good, because every time someone died (which was quite often) I found it brought me down and rammed home the reality of my situation.

Lynn said to think about the benefits of going, giving myself something to get out of bed for and spending time with people in my situation. She and Nikki also arranged for me to attend the Lewis-Manning Hospice as a day patient. I was to return to the Day Centre on a Monday and begin attending Lewis-Manning on a Thursday.

Lewis-Manning is more structured than the Day Centre, they run a sixteen week program focussed on a Wheel of Life exercise, where they support you to look at your life and find ways to make it more balanced. Like the Day Centre, there is the opportunity to do art and craft projects or sit around and chat with others, but they also offer a one-to-one chat with a nurse each week.

During my first week at Lewis-Manning I met with Kay (a nurse), who had to do an assessment to ensure I was a suitable candidate for their programme. She asked me what point I felt I was at, and the flood gates opened again. Talking to her, I couldn't understand why I was even considering starting another cycle of the Capecitabine before seeing Dr Hickish. I had, what I can only describe as a 'light bulb' moment. I didn't want to be having any more treatment. I was done. I always felt I had to keep fighting for the girls, but what good was it, them seeing me laid on the bed or sofa sleeping all the time, or crying as much as I did. It was time to move on, if they were going to keep me alive with drugs, then my life needed to be worthwhile … and at that time it wasn't.

The decision felt empowering, that I was taking control of a situation that had long ago got way out of control. I realised that I was actually in charge of my body and that I could make decisions about what was going to happen to it. I knew it wasn't going to be easy and it was a big responsibility, because it meant the cancer would get me sooner this way and that would affect my whole family, but it also meant that I would have some time, with no drugs involved, to enjoy my family and make some more happy memories. I wanted the girls to remember me as a normal, happy mummy, not someone who sleeps and cries all the time.

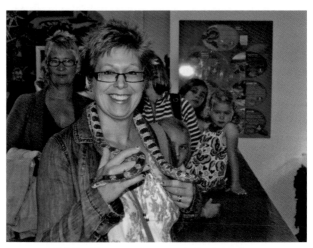

Nikki holding a snake on a visit to Longleat;
something she would never have contemplated before cancer

I spoke to the people closest to me, Kev, Mum and Dad, Mel and Matt, and my friends Cathy, Rhea and Keren. They all said they would support me whatever I decided, they all assured me that I wasn't letting anyone down (which had been playing on my mind), but they all said, "See what Dr Hickish has to say." They were all still hoping that Dr Hickish would come up with something else. I humoured them and agreed to keep an open mind, but I knew I had made up my mind.

When I did see Dr Hickish, he told me that he could reduce the dose of the Capecitabine, or give me a longer break, but I stuck to my guns and told him I had made my decision, I couldn't stay on these drugs. He told me he understood and that some people do struggle to cope with the side effects of different drugs. He went on to say that I could, however, stay on the Lapatinib. It wouldn't work as well or for as long on its own, but it was still worth continuing with it. He then went on to say that when the Lapatinib does stop working, there are other drug options. I didn't feel I had the opportunity to say I had decided enough was enough and I didn't want to try other options. I came out of the appointment feeling somewhat bamboozled. Over the past few days I had made a massive decision, started to get my head around letting nature take its course and expediting my death, and now I was back in limbo.

30

Deep depression

It didn't take long for me to be feeling better physically, but emotionally I really struggled. I couldn't get my head around what I wanted to happen, but I couldn't accept the idea of just going with the flow and seeing what happened. After seeing Dr Hickish I spent the next three days in tears. I felt that I'd let myself down by not telling him how I felt about treatment, I felt drained at the idea of having to live like this for longer than I had already and I felt frustrated that I couldn't just enjoy feeling better in myself, enjoy being awake and not being sick.

On the third day I went out with Cathy. We had a deal for use of a hotel's leisure facilities and then lunch. Swimming is something I have always enjoyed and something Cathy and I had been used to doing a lot together since we were teenagers. Depending on whether we were on a fitness drive or not would determine the strenuousness of the swimming; sometimes we would just plod up and down the pool, chatting as we went, other times we would do quick bursts of ten lengths at a time, then have a break and a chat, before ten more lengths, and so on. On this occasion I couldn't even be bothered to put my swimsuit on, so just sat on a lounger watching Cathy swim and blinking back the tears.

Over lunch I cried several times. I couldn't understand why I couldn't pull myself together; staying on the Lapatinib was a positive thing, and if I felt stronger physically then perhaps when the time came I would feel able to consider the other options that Dr Hickish had mentioned, but I was feeling that life was a chore and stopping treatment had seemed like an easy way out. Cathy told me I needed to speak to my GP for extra support in coping. She said I couldn't live like this and I needed to be able to find joy in everyday life.

The next day I phoned Dr Mitchell; he came out to see me and listened to all I had to say. He told me that he couldn't increase the anti-depressant I was on, because I was taking the maximum dose for someone not in residential psychiatric care, he was also reluctant to try changing my anti-depressant, because that would involve weaning off the current one and then waiting for a new one to take effect. He explained that a new method being used by doctors now is to add a small dose of a different anti-depressant alongside the current one. He prescribed a drug called Sertraline. He then went on to suggest a technique called 'Mindfulness' – despite its roots in centuries old Buddhist Meditation, thanks to Jon Kabat-Zinn, it has become the latest thing in Western psychology:

'Mindfulness means paying attention in a particular way: on purpose, in the present moment, and non-judgmentally. This kind of attention nurtures greater awareness, clarity, and acceptance of present-moment reality.'
Jon Kabat-Zinn (1992)

Dr Mitchell said Mindfulness involved focussing on the present moment, rather than worrying about the past or future. He recommended a book that explained it in more detail and included a CD of mindfulness meditation practices (Mindfulness: A Practical Guide to Finding Peace in a Frantic World by Prof. Mark Williams and Danny Penman 2011). He emphasised the importance of giving it a real try and committing to the time required to do it properly.

I ordered the book, keen to get stuck in. However, when it arrived I soon realised I was going to struggle to take it seriously, and the time required for the meditations – fifteen minutes each morning and again at night, seven days a week – felt daunting. The morning meditations during the week weren't a problem, but if Kev was at home in the evenings, I couldn't do it. Our flat isn't big enough for me to be able to shut myself away without being disturbed – meaning the weekends were also impossible. Although the concept made sense to me, I just couldn't put it into practice.

The book suggested doing everyday tasks, such as tooth brushing or eating, 'mindfully'. On the rare occasion I remembered to brush my teeth mindfully, I couldn't see how it was going to help me enjoy day to day life and feel strong enough to cope with mundane chores. I'm sorry to say that after about a week I gave up.

I found that physically I was functioning well; we took part in another Race for Life, which I completed on foot. I was doing the school runs – both ways, and doing things with the girls at weekends. The weather over the summer was lovely, so we spent a lot of time on the beach, but I often felt I was going through the motions. I worried about all sorts of silly things, actually it was more than worrying, more like obsessing – Christmas, how we were going to afford it, what we were going to buy, how we were going to afford to finish the work on the flat, etc. I also experienced anxiety, feeling panicky if Kev suggested doing something slightly spontaneous. Nikki told me that the anxiety and stress was probably a result of starting another anti-depressant and it would pass once my body gets used to the new drug. She was right, after a couple of weeks it had all passed.

So physically I was feeling better, I was no longer suffering anxiety, but I still couldn't motivate myself to do anything, I had lost interest in everything that I used to enjoy, I didn't read, I didn't write in my diary, I sat in front of mind-numbing television, or worse, on some days I just sat on the sofa gazing into space – hours would pass like that.

When I spoke to the nurses at Lewis-Manning they tried so hard to encourage me, but everything they suggested – helping out at the girls' school, volunteering in a charity shop, etc., just seemed like too much hard work and didn't interest me. I found it frustrating that when the girls were around I could do things with them, but when I was on my own I felt I had no purpose.

One day at Lewis-Manning, Sally, the Day Hospice Manager asked me if I would mind having a chat with Rachel Lapworth, Director of Development, as she was considering new ideas for publicity. Rachel told me that I was currently Lewis-Manning's youngest patient and asked me whether I would mind having my photo taken to be used for publicity, particularly in trying to change people's perceptions that hospices are somewhere for old people to go and die.

Rachel and I chatted and she told me lots about the different work the hospice does. I soon realised that the day hospice was a small part of what goes on. Rachel asked me what sort of things I enjoy doing. I told her how I hadn't felt much like doing anything lately, but how I used to really enjoy writing and would love to get back into it. Her eyes lit up as she told me about a new community project the hospice was running called 'Women Inspiring Women'. It involved women talking about their lives and experiences to inspire other women, to encourage women to realise that they have wisdom and knowledge that can help other women. She told me that she'd had the idea of interviewing staff and patients of the hospice, asking them to talk about their greatest love, their precious memories, their greatest achievements, defining moments, biggest surprises, etc. She then asked me if I'd be interested in carrying out these interviews.

I was amazed that as a patient I would be asked to do something like this, and also very excited. Yes, I actually felt excited about something and was very keen to get started. I found it frustrating that I had to wait for letters to go out explaining the project and asking for volunteers, but feeling that first stirring of desire to engage in something, motivated me to go and sit at the art table. Sarah, the creative artist, showed me a little soft dog that she had made. It was incredible, even more incredible when she showed me a lump of fluff and said that was how the dog had started. She explained the art of 'Needle Felting' to me, a technique where barbed needles are used to tangle and compact fibres of wool into a three-dimensional object. She gave me a book to look through to choose what I wanted to make. I couldn't imagine ever being able to create anything from these lumps of fluff, and seeing the intricate designs in the book convinced me further, but Sarah wouldn't take no for an answer and suggested I try a mouse. She showed me what to do and miraculously I created something … admittedly not a mouse, the creature I created began to look more like a rabbit, so we just adapted it.

I felt a real sense of achievement and realised that I could tick 'Try a new craft' off my list of 'Things to do before I'm Forty'.

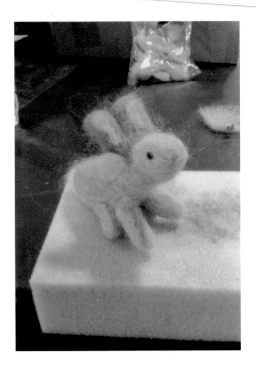

31

A new me

Over the next few weeks I conducted in-depth interviews with three day hospice patients. It was exhausting work, but so interesting and rewarding, I could tell that the subjects were benefitting from the opportunity to talk about their lives, the questions were thought provoking and brought up memories and ideas that they wanted to explore further. I was honoured to be part of their journey of reminiscence and self-discovery and, as Rachel had suggested, I was able to draw out advice from these ladies that would encourage and support other women.

The writing up of the interviews didn't go as smoothly as I'd expected. With the first write-up I did, when I showed it to the lady I'd interviewed, she hated it. She had been brutally honest about certain parts of her life and didn't feel comfortable seeing it in black and white and knowing that others may see it. I had to heavily edit it, which I felt took away the essence of what had been said and what she had been through. It made me sad that so much had to be censored to protect other people.

The second subject sadly passed away before I was able to complete her write-up and I felt it was inappropriate to continue. In fact, having done the interviews and drawn out messages of encouragement, I then felt the rest of the interviews weren't actually that beneficial. Rachel agreed, and with that twinkle in her eye said, "As long as they have served a purpose ... and you never know what it might lead to." I wondered then if the purpose they had served was to get me interested in something again and involved in something worthwhile.

As for what it led to ... in October, as part of Breast Cancer Awareness month, Lewis-Manning held a ladies' lunch called 'Celebrating Women'. Rachel asked me if I would like to speak at the lunch. The thought terrified me, but I said, "Yes." (After all, this was a year of opportunities and new experiences.)

Back at university, when I used to smoke, I didn't tend to have a cigarette until at least lunchtime, more often dinner time, but on days when I had to do a presentation to the class, usually as part of an assessment, Rhea would find me in the kitchen having a cigarette instead of toast for breakfast; the first of several cigarettes before the dreaded moment that I would have to stand in front of my classmates and deliver my presentation. My legs would be like jelly, my mouth would go dry and I would speak way too fast. Yet here I was agreeing to speak about my experiences living with cancer to a group of seventy women whom I had never met before. Was I mad?

Rachel was very clear that it was my decision, that I could change my mind at any time – even on the day of the lunch if I wanted, as they had something else they could use on standby. That knowledge helped me feel more relaxed, but I was determined to do it.

As I sat at my laptop trying to find the words I wanted to use to articulate what it is actually like to be living with breast cancer, I reflected on the past five years and all that I'd been through and this reinforced to me the reason why I so wanted to do the talk. The person I was before cancer would have been reluctant to do the talk, the person I'd been over the past few months would never have been able to do the talk, but this was a new phase of my life, the new me needed new challenges and this was going to be a character building experience.

I was first on the programme and was pleased to be getting it out of the way early on. It went well; I was nervous, but manageably so. The ladies laughed in the right places and you could hear a pin drop at other times. When I'd finished I gratefully accepted a large glass of wine. Throughout the rest of the lunch I had many compliments and I went home feeling proud of myself. I had achieved something that only weeks before would have been impossible to imagine.

The talk at the ladies lunch led to other opportunities; a few weeks later Lewis-Manning held their annual End of Life Conference, this year titled 'Death into Dying'. The conference was for professional people involved in the death process, and focussed on the social aspects of death and how to utilise natural support networks. I was first to talk, to give a patient's perspective. I used the same speech as before and again it was well received; in the break I was given lots of compliments. I stayed for the rest of the conference, finding it all very interesting. Lynn (CNN) was one of the delegates and told me that when she saw me standing up on the podium, she just couldn't believe it was the same person she had seen such a short time ago, crying about how awful things were and wanting to die – I couldn't really believe it either.

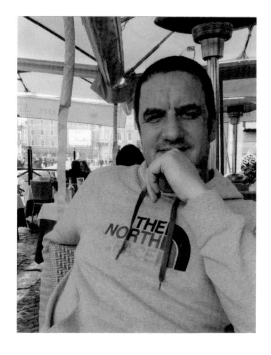

Nikki started a Facebook '100 happy days' blog on January 22nd 2014, and Kev featured on May 1st (Day 100) with Nikki's caption:

'He's waited 99 days for this! It may be cheesy & soppy, but for me happiness is having Kevin by my side everyday through thick & thin. He may not be perfect, but he's perfect for me!'

As I was feeling so much better I decided to get to work on my 'Things to do before I'm Forty' list. I looked at theatre listings and booked to see *The Vagina Monologues* with Mum, and *Evita* with Clare, who I used to work with, and her daughter.

Mum and I heard that Paloma Faith was coming to Bournemouth; we both loved her music, so excitedly looked into booking tickets. We were disappointed to discover that the show was sold out. I continued to Google to see if she was appearing anywhere else near to us, and nothing really came up until I spotted an advert by a Bournemouth hotel offering dinner, bed and breakfast and tickets to the concert. It seemed extravagant, but Wow! what a treat it would be. We booked the tickets, and when the time came we thoroughly enjoyed ourselves. We shopped during the day, and it was so nice to leave what had been a fantastic concert and just walk across the road. We sat in the bar for a drink before going to bed and then woke up to a beautiful sea view. Perfect!

Things were really going well for me and continued to do so. The Lewis-Manning conference had been sponsored by local funeral director and bereavement service, Chester Pearce. The managing director, Stephen Nimmo, had also spoken at the conference about a programme that his organisation had developed as a result of the previous year's conference. 'CHOICES' came about because delegates had expressed a need for a more 'joined up thinking to bring greater comfort to those facing the end of their lives'. Volunteers are trained to be better communicators with the dying and are available through hospices, hospitals, care homes and patients' own homes, to talk about all aspects of death – from the process of dying and where they want to be when they die, to funeral plans and will making.

Stephen's company had also recently developed an idea, which came about following a conversation he'd had with his nine year old stepson. They'd been walking in a cemetery and Taylor observed that the gravestones didn't give much information about the person who had died. He said he wanted to know if that man had any brothers or sisters and what he did for a job. Stephen thought about this and wondered if this was something other people would want. He came up with the idea of putting QR codes (from Quick Response code, a 2d bar code used to provide access to information through a smartphone) on to grave stones and other memorials, with a link to website information about the deceased, either created by the person before their death or by the family afterwards.

Stephen was involved in creating a QR memorial for victims of the Titanic disaster in Southampton. This story was picked up by local news and, subsequently, BBC's *The One Show*. Stephen was asked if he would be interested in doing a piece about the QR memorials for The One Show. He agreed and thought of me. He'd heard me at the conference talking about my work with the adoption service and my understanding of how important it is for people to understand their roots and how, because of this, I had created memory books for my children following my diagnosis. Stephen felt this would be a relevant way to back up what he is doing and a nice way of humanising the topic. I immediately agreed, it sounded really interesting – and after all, I had to jump at every opportunity offered to me.

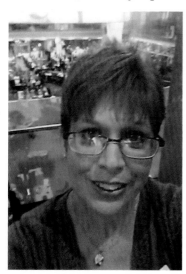

Nikki (selfie) at the BBC on the day that her interview went on air

One cold, but sunny February morning, the BBC filmed Stephen at his stone mason's, and then came to film with me at the hospice. Ex Radio 1 DJ, Andy Kershaw, interviewed me. We chatted about what I had done for the girls, and why. We talked about what could be included on a QR memorial if you should want to do one, and we talked about whether the idea would really hit off or if it were just a bit of a gimmick.

We chatted for well over an hour, for what would ultimately become a five minute slot on the programme. It was fascinating seeing how it was done, and I must admit to developing a bit of a girly crush on Andy Kershaw. I was pleased I waited until after the filming to Google him, as I don't think I would have felt anywhere near as relaxed with him had I realised just how famous he is.

Doing the interview and thinking about how passionate I had become about the idea of life histories being left for future generations, I began to wonder if this was an idea I could develop further – some way of encouraging people (and not just ill people) to create some sort of legacy so that their children and grandchildren would know all about where they came from.

32

The 40th birthday party we thought she would never see

Here the narrative is taken up by Nikki's mum, Ann Carter ...

We tentatively planned Nic's 40th birthday party. What would the theme be? One of her friends had already had an 80's party and Nic was unsure as to what her's would be; it could be Bucking Broncos, it could be James Bond characters, it could be ... ? In the end she settled for 'Glitz and Glamour – dress to impress'.

She ordered her dress ... full length, covered in blue sequins, with the highest heels you could imagine ... 'killer heels'!

We booked the hall; the same one where we had held her wedding reception and her first 'farewell' party, when she was 35.

Her 40th birthday party was held in the evening on the Sunday of May Bank Holiday weekend, so we shopped for food on the Saturday and spent all day Sunday preparing food and titivating ourselves.

We had to keep secret the fact that a limousine had been booked, and this wasn't that easy as Nic was trying to organize, as usual!

I went with her dad and decorated the hall, then stayed there, awaiting the cake (kindly baked and decorated by her Lewis-Manning friends) and the DJ.

People began to arrive and it was obvious that everyone had made the glitz and glamour effort; there were sparkles galore and some very suave-looking young men. Finally, the limo turned into the drive and, wow, she looked sensational as she emerged from the car with her lovely family and friends.

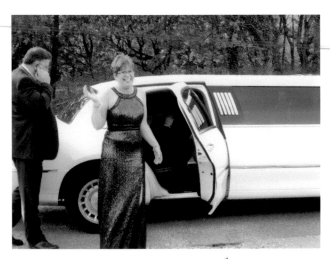

Nikki emerging from the limousine, 4th May 2014

An amazing evening followed, and Leah and Megan came back and stayed with us afterwards, so that Nic would not be woken too early in the morning. She had had a wonderful time, received lots of beautiful cards and presents, and had been surrounded by all those who loved her best.

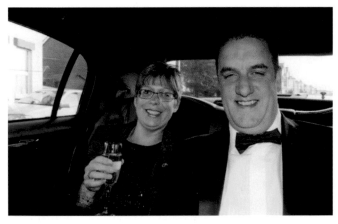

Nikki and Kev in the limo, going home from the party

She had ticked off lots of things from her 'bucket list':

- See a show – we saw The Vagina Monologues and she saw Evita
- Go to a concert – we went to Paloma Faith at the BIC
- Ride a horse – she rode a horse in Weymouth
- Try a new spa treatment – she tried Garra Ruffa
- Finish my book and get on the route to publishing – nearly!
- Visit a new city – she and Kev visited Rome
- Paint a picture – she painted a landscape, which is in her bedroom
- Wear a pair of killer heels – she wore them to her party
- Try a new craft – she tried needle felting at Lewis-Manning
- Volunteer – helping at school
- Karaoke – oh yes, we went to a karaoke bar!

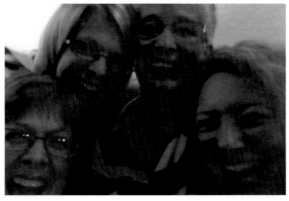

Nikki, Mel, Ann (Mum) and Cathy - selfie at the Karaoke Night, 2014

Together with her friend Rhea, Nic, Leah and Megan had tickets to see One Direction at Wembley on June 8th. The date was fast approaching and there was great excitement, with the days being counted down.

It had become noticeable that Nic was taking longer to get over exerting days and she was having to rest more. She was also feeling very nauseous and suffering from upset tummies quite often. On Friday, May 30th, Nic went to her GP and was diagnosed with a suspected kidney infection. She was prescribed anti-biotics and sent on her way. Over the weekend her condition did not improve and we were glad that she had a pre-chemo appointment on the Monday.

When she arrived at the hospital, however, she collapsed in the car park. I got her up to Ward 10 and she was examined by the doctor, who felt she should be admitted to Poole Hospital. At Poole they seemed quite confident that she would become fit enough to go to the concert on the following Sunday, as, at that time that was her main concern. However, it became apparent that she did not have an infection and that her kidney was blocked. A scan showed glandular enlargement, although no one would confirm it was the cancer.

After having a litre and a half of fluid drained from her chest cavity, she was transferred to Bournemouth Hospital, where she had a stent inserted in her kidney. She became quite distressed at Bournemouth Hospital, because the surgical ward did not seem to appreciate the amount of morphine she needed to control her pain, and as soon as she was able, she discharged herself in order to self-medicate her pain relief at home.

We were having a barbecue for Leo's 7th birthday, and she came to our house with Kev and the girls. Although she stayed indoors, she was glad to be surrounded by her family again.

Obviously, there was no way she was going to be able to go to Wembley, so Kev took the girls to meet Rhea and her family, and they took them into the concert, while I stayed with Nic and we watched Dirty Dancing on the TV. By the Wednesday of that week, we felt the need to call her GP out. He examined her, but said that, as she had an appointment on Ward 10 the next day, he was happy to leave her at home. During the afternoon, however, she deteriorated quite rapidly. We called an ambulance and she was re-admitted to Poole Hospital.

Dr Hickish came to talk to Nic, Kev and myself, and he explained that it was Nic's liver that was causing so much discomfort. He also confirmed that there was now no treatment which would give any lasting benefit; the only thing was to admit her to the Macmillan Unit at Christchurch Hospital, where they would be able to manage her pain and keep her comfortable for some time.

Nic passed away at 9:15am on Wednesday 25th June 2014.

33

A tribute to Nic

Narrative by Ann ...

When Nic was admitted to the Macmillan Unit and she knew that she did not have long to live, we discussed her funeral arrangements again; they had obviously changed as Leah and Megan were now of an age to understand what was happening and wanted to be involved with all that was going on.

Uncle Steve had a penchant for writing personal poetry, he had written lots of poems for friends and family on different occasions and Nic asked him if he felt he would be able to write a poem for her funeral. He has obviously known Nic very well since she was a baby, and this is the beautiful poem he wrote, which sums up the essence of our lovely daughter and managed to bring smiles and laughter on a day of unbearable sadness.

'Nic' *by Uncle Steve*

The day that Nic came into this world,
her parents were so very proud
A beautiful bouncing baby,
all cuddly, but boy was she loud.

Farleys and milk just weren't enough,
for Nic in her baby phase
She decided one day to eat a snail,
there was slime on her face for days

Always so fond of eating,
Nic saved the best bits till last
That way the tastiest portion
doesn't disappear too fast.

While dining with Granddad Carter,
Nic was given some chocolate cake
A huge chocolate button sat on it
she moved it to the side of the plate.

Eating slowly as young ladies do,
not wanting to appear a glutton
She turned her back for a moment,
and Matt went and nicked her button.

Al once took Nic to ballet
with her little sister Mel
The weather was foul it was pouring,
the rain just fell and fell.

Just picture those two little angels
all cute in their best ballet suits
Picture their tight fitting leotards,
and Nic in her wellington boots.

As she went through her teens, she chattered at school,
but constantly aimed for the top
She was pretty and cute and sweet natured,
but prone to the occasional strop.

Nic was a girl with opinions,
outspoken with values and pride
That's what she got from her mother,
and her time in Christchurch Girl Guides.

When she left school she nannied,
and worked for a while in a pub
And then she moved down to Brighton,
a place she would soon come to love.

At Uni she read social science,
and achieved a 2:1 degree
And then she came back to Bournemouth,
to work for the BBC. (Bournemouth Borough Council)

Now we all have ways of making it home,
when we've had a night on the town
Some get a cab, some stagger and sway,
and some people just fall down.

Nic had her own way of doing things,
when she'd had her liquid fill
She got a lift to Chalfont Avenue,
and rolled all the way down the hill.

Then she met Kev and they fell in love,
and married in two thousand and three
And it proved to be as perfect a match,
as any match could be.

A few years later they were blessed with not one,
but two beautiful little daughters
And Nic just took to motherhood,
like the proverbial duck to water.

Two little girls with cute little curls
and pretty like two little poppies
But just as loud as their mother,
and definitely just as stroppy.

Nic loved all the things that most girls love,
chocolates and chick flicks and pink
And purple and dancing and parties,
and of course the occasional drink.

She was older than most of her cousins,
who loved her and were somewhat in awe
Her nephews and nieces adored her,
but let's be honest what's not to adore.

She was a formidable woman,
she was beautiful, forthright and strong
But then came the diagnosis,
and it all went horribly wrong.

But Nic didn't buckle under
she didn't just wallow and stew
She picked herself up, got on with her life
and took whatever life threw.

She cursed that rotten chemo,
and still she went on to make
Thousands of pounds for charity,
through quiz nights, tombola and cakes.

She tried her hand at painting
and making things out of clay
Cardboard and glue and ribbons,
which the girls still do to this day.

She had a few holidays with Kev and the kids,
stroked dolphins and went to LA
It was clear, of the time she had left,
she wouldn't be wasting a day.

She had a brief brush with stardom,
wrote a blog in the local press
She had her feet rubbed by Sophie,
the Countess of Wessex, no less.

She appeared this year on The One Show,
and talked about bar codes on stones
Which help us remember our loved ones
by using our mobile phones.

She made memory boxes for Leah and Meg,
to keep them in touch with their past
Started scrapbooks for them to keep all their life,
to make those memories last.

She made her granny a scrapbook,
in which all the family appear
And she religiously kept it updated,
with photos and notes every year.

Nic made special friends in her lifetime,
friends who she held very dear
They gave her comfort and much support
as her time was drawing near.

Her bucket list before forty,
she managed to complete just in time
Then she had that lovely party,
and wow did she look fine.

I'm sure that's how most will remember,
that beautiful smiling girl
Surrounded by people who loved her,
the people who made her whole world.

That lovely sparkling dress,
and those heels that made her so tall
Her smile as wide as the ocean,
an image to cherish for all.

Nic – I hope they watch Holby where you're going,
play Bon Jovi and watch Rom Coms too
I hope their curtains are purple,
you wouldn't want orange or blue.

Maybe you'll find Uncle Pete there,
or maybe he'll find you
But be on your best behaviour,
your granddads might both be there too.

You're a truly inspiring lady,
and we all feel greatly blessed
To have shared some time with you in our lives,
Nic you are simply the best.

We're waving you off, but not saying goodbye,
your spirit will always be here
The fun, love and charm that you brought to our lives,
will mean that you always feel near.

Epilogue
by Nikki's mum, Ann

To say the last five and a half years have been an emotional rollercoaster is an understatement; firstly the disbelief that this could happen to our family again so soon after we had lost my brother. I gave up work to help Nic look after the girls, as the chemotherapy affected her so badly she could not cope with two little ones. In one of her darkest moments, Nic asked me whether I wished I had never had her; not for a single moment had that thought crossed my mind. I did not want the pain, nor did I want the girls to suffer, but how could I not have known her, how could I not have had her in my life.

There were times when we were short with each other, arguing about things like the fact that she liked rubber gloves loose and I liked them tight; the fact that I put the milk in the mug with the tea bag still in it; that I did not co-ordinate the clothes pegs! Such stupid trivial things, but this was because we were both exhausted both physically and mentally. How do you get through every day knowing that your daughter is dying?

There were times when Kev found it difficult to cope, and although I struggled with this, it did give me the opportunity to spend many quality moments with Nic – it was some consolation that she always felt she could turn to me.

As a mother, my natural instinct is to protect my children, however old they are; I have been unable to protect my daughter from this disease, but she has allowed me to be with her every step of the way; I will always be grateful to her for that. Along the way we have had good times as well, lots of wonderful quality days out; discovering the therapeutic joy of a hot stone massage with an amazing masseuse; going on stage with the ladyboys, several live shows; spa days and even singing in a Karaoke Bar.

This week, I lost my little girl, as I knew I would. My little family will never be complete again, but in the void that is left will be two of the most amazing little girls, who will have inherited their mummy's attributes, and while Nic has done all she can to ease her girls' pain, they will be our catharses.

Nic, I love you and I will always carry your heart in my heart.

Postscript

Nikki

by Heather Freeman
Team Manager, Adoption and Permanence Team, Bournemouth

I first met Nikki when I interviewed her for a job as a family support practitioner in the Bournemouth Family Placement Team. At the time, it was a combined adoption and fostering team and the job Nikki had applied for was always a very popular one. We had over 60 applications, but eventually whittled them down to about six people to interview, Nikki included.

She did well in the formal part of the interview and in the written exercise, but it was in the group exercise that she really stood out. All of those being interviewed were gathered together in a very small room, with the three interviewers observing, and something topical to discuss – I can't remember now what it was. What I do remember though is how well Nikki handled the situation. In these group situations, some people feel they have to dominate the group by talking lots. Nikki didn't need to do so. She listened, and only contributed when she had something to say – and what she said was clear and to the point. It got her the job. It was the week before she married Kev, and I also remember how organised and calm she was about all of the big changes in her life – a move back to Bournemouth, a new job and marriage.

Initially, Nikki's job was mainly supporting foster carers, for example, sorting equipment out, looking after the children they were caring for to give them a break or attend training. Then, in November 2003, the team split into two separate teams, a fostering team and an adoption team. Nikki had a choice as to which team to join and decided to join the adoption team, which I managed. She was still called a 'family support practitioner', but her role changed as I wanted her to focus on making sure that all

150

of the children we were moving to adoptive families understood why they were moving to a new family. With the older children, this meant direct work, but, as most of the children we were placing were under three years old, I also wanted all of the children being placed for adoption to have a Lifestory book, explaining about their past and keeping memories alive.

There was no similar role anywhere else in the country that we were aware of, so Nikki, methodical as ever, set about doing her research. She read books and articles, spoke to the clinical psychologists who worked closely with us, and met with adoptive parents and youngsters who had been adopted. At the time it was recognised that children should have Lifestory books, but they were not always completed because of other pressures on the children's social workers, who were the ones who usually completed them. Even if they were completed, they were more or less just photo books, which didn't help children to understand why they were being adopted.

These are Nikki's own words about her work. She sent it to me less than a month before she died, as she was due to give a presentation about leaving a personal legacy in the way of memory books for family members when you die, and wanted to use her experience from work to back up her argument.

> *'Before I was ill and retired from work, my job was to prepare children for their move to a new family through adoption. In the past the child's social worker would gather together some photographs of the child's foster care placements and possibly some of their birth family, put them into a photo album with a few facts and other souvenirs and that would be considered sufficient Lifestory work. New research became available evidencing the need for more in-depth work to be done.*
>
> *Childcare experts, Vera Fahlberg, Kate Cairns and Joy Rees, looked at the way a positive early attachment to a primary caregiver and a deeper understanding of their roots helped traumatised children to be more resilient and more able to settle and make new positive attachments. In her book,*

'A Child's Journey Through Placement' (1991) Vera Fahlberg states, 'It is difficult to grow up as a psychologically stable adult if one is denied access to one's own history'.

In light of this research, and when a new post became available within the Bournemouth Adoption Service, my manager asked me to study the research and take over the Lifestory work aspect of the child's move to their new home. I began to do direct work with children, talking about their own memories and helping them to understand why they could no longer live with their foster carer or return to their birth family. The Lifestory book was a by-product of this work – equally important, but not the sole purpose of Lifestory work.

Bournemouth Adoption Service Lifestory work model soon became considered best practice among other local authorities, and at the time I was diagnosed and had to leave I was setting up meetings to discuss my work with Social Workers from other areas.'

Nikki was a valued member of the team on a personal level too and her diagnosis shocked us all. She worked as hard as everyone else, but was the one in the team who looked after herself by having a short lunch break, away from her desk every day. The rest of us just ate at our desks, but Nikki always took her sandwiches into the kitchen with a book, and had half an hour reading or chatting to people.

We were with her through both pregnancies. With both, she had low blood pressure and a couple of times fainted in the staff toilets, so every time she went out of the team room and was gone longer than we expected, someone would check she was OK. She came back to work after her maternity leave both times, and, as we were a very close team, we saw Leah and Megan growing up.

She was devastated when her Uncle Pete became ill and died, and I remember going up to London for a conference with Nikki and 2 other members of the team and her talking about what had happened. At the time, Nikki herself was looking good. She was settled in her work, was establishing a reputation locally and further afield for her pioneering work, Leah and Megan were over the tiny baby stage, and Mel was about to get married. Nikki had been coming into the office with make up on and wearing heels to get used to them for the wedding! She had mentioned twinges in her hip, but put it down to having carried Megan round Legoland a few weeks before.

Then, in the week after Mel's wedding, the devastating diagnosis.

Nikki didn't return to work after she became ill, but always remained one of the team, and joined us for all of our social events. Even people who joined the team after she had left got to know her. But more importantly, she left a legacy in what she started with her Lifestory books and the direct work she did with children. Sue took over her role at work when she left and developed it further, and now there are three full time family support practitioners in the team.

Just before Nikki became ill, we had had Ofsted in to inspect the adoption service and they had been very impressed with what she was doing. They returned in February 2012 and as an adoption service we were rated as outstanding, and again the Lifestory work was commented on. Then in November 2012, we were named as 'Adoption Service of the Year' by the British Association for Adoption and Fostering at an awards ceremony in London hosted by Nicky Campbell. The award was for the work we were doing in preparing children for moves to adoptive families and our Lifestory work – something which Nikki started.

Other adoption services now copy what we do, as we are now seen as leaders in the field. For example, earlier this year, we were contacted and asked to help a voluntary adoption agency, which had been commissioned by the Department for Education to develop a good practice guide on Lifestory work.

Nikki's part in all of this was enormous. She was a pioneer in the field, and her contribution to improving the lives of vulnerable children carries on, even though her own life was tragically cut short. We will always remember her – and miss her.

BOURNEMOUTH ECHO

Wed 3 December 2014 - by Diana Henderson

Tree lights switched on in memory of mum Nikki Hastings

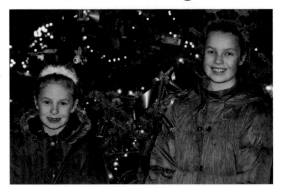

The young daughters of a former Poole hospice patient switched on special tree lights in her memory at a Light Up a Life ceremony.

Nikki Hastings, who became an ambassador for the Lewis-Manning Hospice at Evening Hill, died aged 40 in June after being diagnosed with secondary breast cancer in 2008.

Her daughters, Megan, eight, and Leah, nine, switched on the lights in the hospice grounds in memory of their much-missed Mum.

Nikki, who was a day patient at the hospice, was a former Daily Echo blogger, who regularly shared her story at hospice events, including on the BBC's The One Show earlier in the year.

Initially told she had just months to live, she battled the disease for six years, giving her more time with husband Kevin and her girls.

"We felt extremely privileged that Leah and Megan switched on the Christmas tree lights this year and would like to thank them and their family for helping make it such a special event," said Paul Tucker, Lewis-Manning's communications officer.

Light Up a Life is a time of celebration and reflection to remember the life of a loved one by dedicating a light in their memory.

The annual event was attended by the Mayor of Poole, Cllr Peter Adams, with performances from Daisy Lapworth and Sound of Soul choir.